THE MIGRATION OF SKILLED HEALTH PERSONNEL IN THE PACIFIC REGION

A SUMMARY REPORT

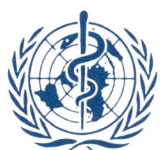

**World Health Organization
Regional Office for the Western Pacific
Manila, Philippines**

WHO Library Cataloguing in Publication Data

The migration of skilled health personnel in the Pacific Region: a summary report.

1. Emigration and immigration 2. Health personnel 3. Pacific islands.

ISBN 92 9061 175 8   (NLM Classification: W 76)

© World Health Organization 2004

All rights reserved.

The designations employed and the presentation of the material in this publication do not imply the expression of any opinion whatsoever on the part of the World Health Organization concerning the legal status of any country, territory, city or area or of its authorities, or concerning the delimitation of its frontiers or boundaries. Dotted lines on maps represent approximate border lines for which there may not yet be full agreement.

The mention of specific companies or of certain manufacturers' products does not imply that they are endorsed or recommended by the World Health Organization in preference to others of a similar nature that are not mentioned. Errors and omissions excepted, the names of proprietary products are distinguished by initial capital letters.

The World Health Organization does not warrant that the information contained in this publication is complete and correct and shall not be liable for any damages incurred as a result of its use.

Publications of the World Health Organization can be obtained from Marketing and Dissemination, World Health Organization, 20 Avenue Appia, 1211 Geneva 27, Switzerland (tel: +41 22 791 2476; fax: +41 22 791 4857; email: bookorders@who.int). Requests for permission to reproduce WHO publications, in part or in whole, or to translate them – whether for sale or for noncommercial distribution – should be addressed to Publications, at the above address (fax: +41 22 791 4806; email: permissions@who.int). For WHO Western Pacific Regional Publications, request for permission to reproduce should be addressed to Publications Office, World Health Organization, Regional Office for the Western Pacific, P.O. Box 2932, 1000, Manila, Philippines, Fax. No. (632) 521-1036, email: publications@wpro.who.int

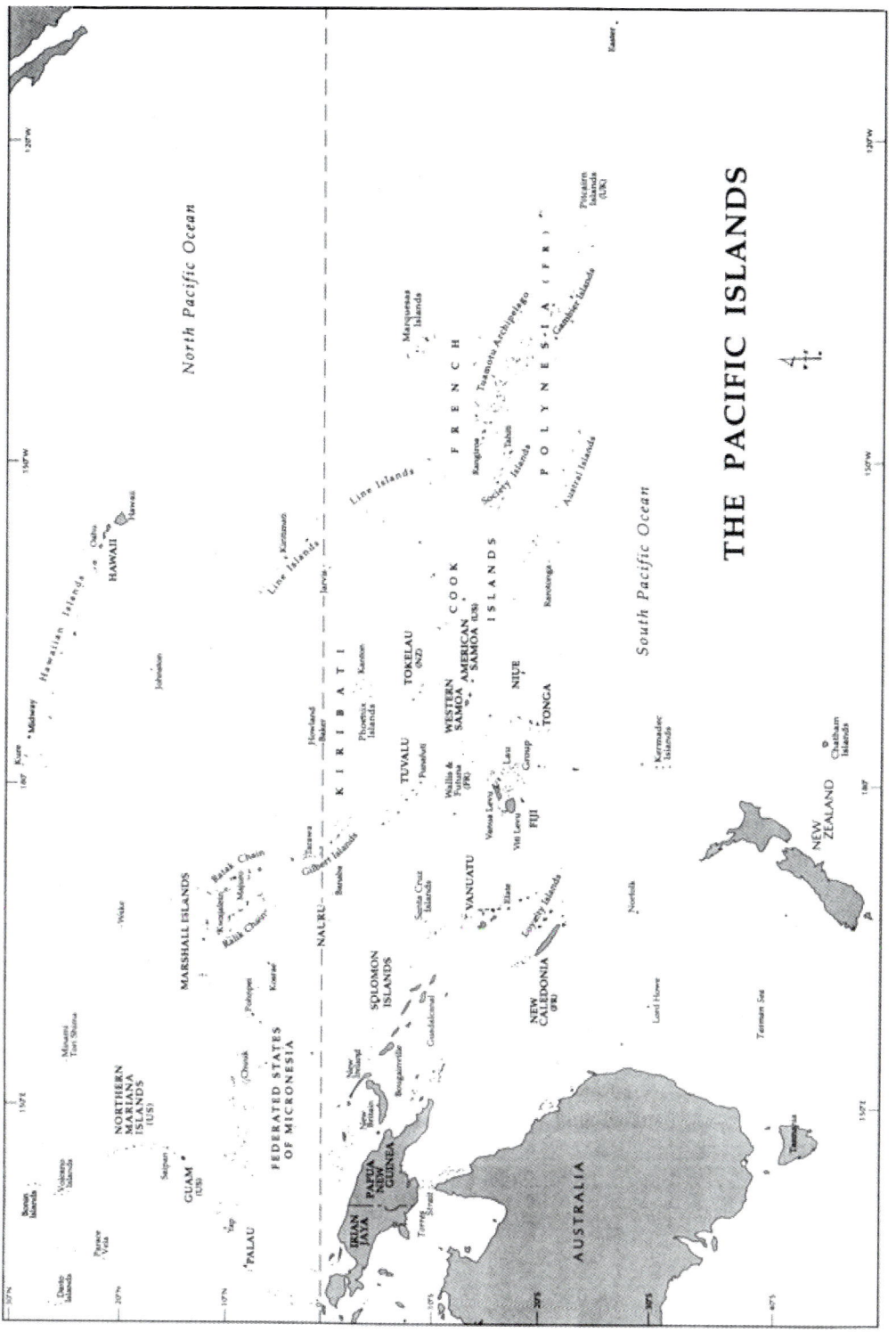

Disclaimer: The boundaries and names shown and the designations used on this map do not imply the expression of an opinion whatsoever on the part of WHO concerning the legal status of any country, territory, city or areas or its authorities.

ACKNOWLEDGEMENTS

Completion of this study was only possible through the leadership of the researcher, Professor John Connell, Head, School of Geosciences, University of Sydney and the commitment and involvement of a large number of different people, including study participants.

We are very grateful to a number of people in several countries for assistance with the data collection, and especially the conducting of questionnaire surveys, most of which were undertaken in late 2000 and early 2001. These include: in Fiji, Dr Taiamoni Tongamoa; in Samoa, Ms Tautalaaso Taulealo and Mr Keneti Vaigafa; in Tonga, Ms Nicole Maron; in Vanuatu, Ms Sarah Naupa; in Palau, Ms Julie Tellei (on behalf of the Palau Resource Institute); in Canada, Dr Charles Greenberg; in New Zealand, Dr Sitaleki Finau; and in Australia, Ms Carmen Voigt-Graf, Ms Paulina Fusitu'a and Ms Alanna Linn. The quantitative data analysis was done under the direction of Associate Professor Richard Brown of the University of Queensland. We are very appreciative of the assistance provided by Amanda Wilkinson in the analysis of qualitative data.

CONTENTS

Acknowledgements iv

Executive summary vii

1. Introduction 1

2. Literature review 5

    2.1 General migration in Pacific island countries 5
    2.2 Island states and the health workforce 10
    2.3 Health 11
    2.4 The human resource context 16

3. Study rationale and methodology 19

4. Findings 23

    4.1 Fiji 23
    4.2 Palau 35
    4.3 Samoa 38
    4.4 Tonga 43
    4.5 Vanuatu 51
    4.6 Intentions to migrate 52
    4.7 Trainees 55

5. Discussion 57

    5.1 Structural context 57
    5.2 Survey 59

6. Conclusions 63

7. Future directions 67

References 71

Tables

Table 1:	Pacific populations	10
Table 2:	Intention to migrate model: Descriptive statistics	53
Table 3:	Probit regression model results	54

Appendices

Appendix 1: Sample survey questionnaire 75
Appendix 2: Newspaper articles 93

EXECUTIVE SUMMARY

Migration of health professionals in Pacific island countries and areas is a growing and significant concern in regards to the provision of health services and the quality of life for various small and scattered population groups. Over the past two decades there has been a widespread loss of skilled health professionals (SHPs) in most independent Pacific island countries, through emigration, mainly to metropolitan states. Skilled migration has occurred in a wider context of emigration, part of the creation of a 'transnational community of kin' and significant for the flow of remittances to island states where economic growth has been limited. The loss of SHPs has come at a cost to island states and health systems because of the high costs of training and the reduction in the effectiveness of health care.

A survey of 280 migrant and non-migrant SHPs in key countries within the Pacific – Tonga, Samoa, Fiji, Palau and Vanuatu – and in metropolitan destinations, examined the rationale for migration. There is extraordinary consistency in general explanation of migration. Within and beyond the Pacific, these focus on low remuneration, inflexible hours, the lack of continuing educational opportunities, limited training facilities, shortages of supplies and equipment and a poor working environment, especially in rural and remote areas (where health needs are least well served). In a context where mobility (and emigration) is often the norm, governments have rarely sought to discourage it, relatives are increasingly likely to be overseas and public spending cuts are systemic. Political instability is a factor in Fiji. However, social and demographic variables are of enormous significance, especially for those who remain in place. The situation is most serious for doctors, especially young and good ones, and more serious in the smaller states. The emigration rates for nurses are steadily increasing as overseas recruitment occurs. More parts of the Pacific are now being affected by skilled emigration.

Migration is not merely an overspill of surplus population, but a definite loss. Migration has clear negative outcomes on both the financial and health systems, limiting progress towards 'Healthy Islands',[1] and possibly even resulting in a regression in that status. Return migration is of limited significance. High levels of migration have contributed to low productivity, poor morale and frustration. All the factors that have stimulated recent migration remain in place. Emigration is likely to continue, while recruitment within the Pacific from outside may increase, and exacerbate the existing situation. The most serious problems of labour shortages are in the smaller states, where skilled human resources are fewer, and in more remote regions.

---

[1] Healthy Islands aims to improve the health and quality of life of people in Pacific countries and areas. This healthy settings approach involves continuously identifying and resolving priority issues related to health, development and well-being by advocating, facilitating and enabling these issues to be addressed in partnerships among communities, organizations and agencies at local, national and regional levels.

Policies to reduce emigration must focus on more appropriate hiring, salary and career structures, more effective in-country training, improved working conditions and incentives (such as part-time private practice and educational benefits for children), continuing professional education, and regulatory and administrative arrangements for recruitment or hiring of health professionals between countries.

1 INTRODUCTION

The most important resource in any small state is its people. The role of human resources is central to development in many small states and the limited availability of skilled human resources can be a constraint to development. Human capital is a critical element in the economic and social development of all societies. In essence, this refers to the 'quality' of human beings; an educated person is likely to yield higher social returns than a less educated person. Equally, someone who is in good health will be a more valuable member of society than someone who is sick.

In the health arena, the significance of human resources is doubled; skilled health personnel directly improve the quality of life for others, who are then able to contribute more to the wider society. Conversely, the lack of availability of skilled health workers has serious implications for the rest of society. This report examines one particular aspect of that availability: the role of migration in the changing distribution of skilled populations.

Tertiary education and training are needed to provide the capacity for continued human resource development in small states, and to generate the skills for analysis, production and maintenance, problem solving and management at both general and specific levels. Access to tertiary education and health professional training are restricted in some small states. In the smallest of them, there is some continued degree of dependence on expatriate technical assistance, often to fill the higher-level positions in the public service (and in the private sector). This situation has only slowly changed.

In most island states there is a continued need to ensure that training and education is relevant to the particular situation of small states. This usually means that it should be more appropriate to meet particular local constraints and requirements. It has been argued that, in general, this has been better achieved in the Caribbean than in the Pacific because of a lack of resources in the latter group of countries to make appropriate curriculum changes (Commonwealth Secretariat, 1997: 130). Hence training within the Pacific region has not necessarily been able to produce either adequate numbers of skilled health personnel or enough people with appropriate skills. This has meant that several countries lack adequate numbers of appropriately skilled health workers.

A constant source of concern in most parts of the Pacific island region is the need for institutional strengthening. First, this means that there should be appropriate facilities to develop adequate numbers of appropriately skilled people within the region. Second, it means ensuring that skilled people remain in place within the region and deliver adequate services. In many island states, the inadequate delivery of services (whether health, education, transport, etc.) has been seen as one of the most substantial constraints to development, and particularly to long-term human resources development. These issues are particularly serious in the smallest states because of the special issue of providing training at high cost for very small numbers of people.

These problems are exacerbated, and usually again most obviously in the smallest states, where there is migration (and thus attrition) of the labour force. This may be significant both within countries, with movement from peripheries (or the unwillingness of skilled personnel to be located there), and between countries, through emigration. Migration of skilled workers has already had a significant impact on the Pacific region.

Migration of skilled health professionals (SHPs) into, within and from the Pacific island countries and areas (PICs) is widely considered to be a growing problem. It is certainly growing in significance. Loss of significant numbers of key health workers affects core national strategies for health sector development, creating problems for health care and for human resource planning and development. This can be a costly loss of scarce and expensively trained human capital. Training of SHPs is particularly costly because of the long duration, the high costs of teaching materials and techniques (and the need for postgraduate education and training programmes). Consequently the loss of SHPs is unusually costly. Replacements may also be costly (and may be lacking in appropriate skills, languages and cultural sensitivity), while ensuring their adequacy, even in terms of their formal qualifications, may be difficult. This creates potential problems in satisfying basic needs, achieving sustainable health strategies and developing healthy islands.

The structural weaknesses of health systems within the PICs have become more evident as the demand for improved health care provision has grown. Improvements in health management are required to ensure that existing resources are used more effectively, through strengthening national capacity to meet management requirements at a national and regional level. This will also lead to addressing the long-term needs of the workforce, and developing a health training and development strategy that meets local needs. This is likely to become more critical with the epidemiological transition from infectious diseases to noncommunicable diseases.

A number of studies have been undertaken by various organizations and individuals but have provided limited, incomplete (and sometimes anecdotal rather than analytical) information on health worker migration and its impacts. There have been no studies of in-migrant SHPs in the region (and very little information on their role). Overall no comprehensive study has been undertaken of the migration of SHPs in PICs within the context of regional (even global) labour markets. Consequently there is inadequate information on the rationale and impacts of the migration of SHPs, or the particular forms of migrant selectivity, in individual countries or in the region as a whole.

Despite the limited amount of good data there is a widespread assumption that the problem of health worker migration is worsening. Indeed there is now even some competition for SHPs between PICs and the view held is that the situation is most acute in the smaller independent states. One dramatic example of this was the observation in a recent report by a Pacific island doctor who noted that as soon as a new doctor arrived in the small island state of Tokelau, there was already "a need to create a good incentive package to prevent this new doctor from leaving to neighbouring countries" (Taitai, 1999: 39). Presumptions of future migration are well entrenched.

The evidence that is available points to some worsening of the situation, in terms of attrition and migration rates, during the last decade. That has accompanied the widespread downsizing (or stabilizing) of civil servant numbers. In turn, that is linked to stagnant economic growth and growing pressure on PICs to engage in comprehensive restructuring. Moreover that situation was already a source of concern a decade ago: "The region faces a crisis in terms of its health work force, not only in terms of direct care providers but at all levels of the system. It is not surprising that one of the most frequently mentioned topics is the shortage of doctors. The physician shortage is only the tip of the iceberg. Inefficiency in health systems is a major problem and there is a crucial need for trained administrative personnel" (Lewis, 1990: 84). It is in this deteriorating context that the study was undertaken.

In some respects these issues are a function of other related problems in PICs: shortages of financial resources; inadequate government commitment to health despite the linkage between poor health and slower economic growth; weak management capacity; and few economies of scale (that contribute to shortages of drugs and technology, alongside human resources). This is also linked to a dependence on offshore facilities (such as education and training facilities and specialist hospitals) especially in scattered islands in PICs, alongside rising expectations for the delivery of services and standards of living. In some places this has led to an emphasis on high technology (and in hospitals) rather than on appropriate technology or the achievement of a balanced workforce. In some contexts there is a weakness in governance and political will (involving organization and commitment at all levels), a lack of interest in the health sector as a place of employment and, more generally, the lack of a 'stakeholder society'. Consequently, there are both long-standing and relatively new constraints to developing a more responsive and appropriate health care system, and there is a real need for this to be addressed quickly.

In response to the trends and problems indicated above, the study, commissioned by the World Health Organization (WHO), set out to evaluate the obstacles to maintaining and improving the quality of health care and health care institutions by examining the scale and impact of high rates of immigration and out-migration of skilled health professionals in PICs. The secondary aim was to develop policies that would minimize the negative impacts of migration.

The initial part of this report reviews the available literature and the surveys of health worker (and other skilled) migration in the Pacific region. This is linked to an examination of recent changes in the stock of health workers in PICs, with particular reference to emigration and immigration, and the impact of these changes on health care provision. The second part of the report reviews the data derived from surveys undertaken in a number of PICs and destination nations, on potential and actual migrants, presently or formerly employed in health care, that focus on the rationale and context for out-migration, and the potential for return migration (of SHPs currently overseas). This is linked to studies of immigrant SHPs in PICs, to examine their migration and employment history and their contribution to the maintenance and improvement of health care in the region. Finally this is reviewed in the context of existing policies that seek to influence the retention, and appropriate allocation of health workers, in PICs, and the potential for developing more effective policies.

In those states that retain a close political tie with a metropolitan nation, including American Samoa, Guam and the Commonwealth of the Northern Marianas (with the United States of America) and French Polynesia, New Caledonia and Wallis and Futuna (with France), the availability of SHPs appears to be better than that in other PICs (in part because salaries and working conditions are superior). This study therefore focuses on those PICs where particular problems have been identified. These primarily include Fiji, Tonga, Samoa, Palau and Vanuatu, but some reference is made to other states in the region where similar issues have been identified. Destinations include New Zealand, Canada, Australia and the United States of America.

A necessary preliminary to the proposed study will be a systematic review of existing studies of the migration of health personnel in the region, other studies of skilled labour migration in PICs (and in similar Caribbean island states) and national development plans and health and human resource plans (where these exist) to seek to determine:

(1) where the migration of SHPs constitutes a particular problem in terms of health, social, economic or other impacts;

(2) if migration is considered to be particularly significant among some categories of health workers;

(3) where countries have adopted specific policies, and with what success, to minimize the impact of migration;

(4) what legislation is in place regarding the licensing of immigrants to practice and the assessment of qualifications; and

(5) what are the presently known socioeconomic and institutional correlates of out-migration of SHPs (with particular reference to age, sex, economic status, qualifications, etc.).

There has been no previous detailed study of the migration of SHPs in this or any other developing island region. Hence this study is likely to have important implications for other countries and regions, especially other island realms, in contributing to more sustainable health care systems.

2
LITERATURE REVIEW

2.1 GENERAL MIGRATION IN PACIFIC ISLAND COUNTRIES

Since the 1960s, there has been a very substantial rise in the extent and significance of migration within and from the Pacific island countries, resulting in absolute population reductions in some of the smallest states. International migration to the metropolitan states on the fringes of the region was initially primarily a Polynesian phenomenon. Many people from Niue, Cook Islands, Tonga, Samoa and American Samoa have moved to New Zealand (from which some have gone on to Australia). Increasingly, as the New Zealand economy has stagnated and immigration restrictions tightened, many have gone to the United States of America. For the smallest states, including Cook Islands, Niue and Tokelau, migration has been particularly dramatic since a very substantial majority of their populations now live overseas, mainly in New Zealand.

In the largest countries of Melanesia, emigration has been relatively insignificant; the larger countries are independent rather than associated states (hence their citizens have more difficulty meeting stringent immigration controls), their economies are more viable and, in some cases, they have fewer skilled personnel (who would meet immigration requirements elsewhere). However, there has long been a significant migration stream, of Fiji-Indians from Fiji, who have gone to several metropolitan destinations, including Australia, New Zealand, Canada and the United States of America. In terms of the migration of SHPs this is the most important stream in the region.

In the last decade especially there has been a very considerable movement of Micronesians from the Marshall Islands and the Federated States of Micronesia particularly to the United States of America, and to its Territories (particularly Guam and the Northern Marianas). Political status has been a significant influence on migration in that the nationals of Cook Islands, Niue and Tokelau are New Zealand citizens and may move there freely, while the nationals of the Federated States of Micronesia, the Marshall Islands and Palau (following the various Compacts of Free Association) are free to migrate to the United States of America and its dependencies. Though there are some regional movements within the Pacific (for example from Wallis and Futuna to New Caledonia), these are usually of lesser volume and consequence.

International movements have been paralleled by intensified migration within particular countries. The migration from remote islands and isolated rural areas to more accessible coastal locations, particularly to urban areas, has grown considerably in recent years. Thus national populations have become increasingly concentrated on the more central urbanized islands, such as Tongatapu in Tonga, Upolu in Samoa, South Tarawa in Kiribati and Efate in Vanuatu. This has tended to accentuate problems of service delivery in remote areas. This situation has in turn accentuated and accounted for some of that movement away from isolated areas.

While the scale of international migration is affected by the vicissitudes of the international economy (but more particularly through the relationship between economic performance in different destinations), migration is primarily affected by uneven development: inequalities, both real and perceived, in socioeconomic opportunities. These include income levels and the desire for access to education and health services. Tertiary education is usually undertaken outside the home country, especially in the smaller states, a factor contributing to emigration (e.g. Workman et al., 1981). Traditionally, metropolitan countries have been the main destinations for tertiary studies, but, as in the case of Cook Islands, the growth of facilities within the Pacific, especially associated with the University of the South Pacific (USP) in Fiji, and the availability of scholarships elsewhere, has both diversified the range of migration options and encouraged new tertiary movements within the Pacific.

It is not possible to identify the extent to which either SHPs are a significant and rising proportion of either emigrants from PICs or immigrants from PICs to metropolitan states, since migration data are too crude or are unavailable, and there is a general unwillingness on the part of both sending and receiving countries to acknowledge the flows of skilled labour (Iredale 2000). There is, however, some indication that skilled workers in general, and SHPs in particular, are a higher proportion of immigrants from PICs to metropolitan states because of the increased focus on skilled migration (within declining immigration numbers) in most destinations, and the continued (and increasing) demand for health workers there. Each of the principal destinations for SHPs – the United States of America, Canada, Australia, New Zealand and the United Kingdom of Great Britain and Northern Ireland – have the acquisition of permanent skilled migrants as one of the objectives of their immigration policies. Indeed, they have become competitors in trying to attract highly skilled (and entrepreneurial) migrants (Cobb-Clark and Connelly 1997). Ironically, many of these migrant's skills were unused because their qualifications, despite contributing to gaining them entry, were unrecognized in the destination.

Migration is both a catalyst and a consequence of social and economic change, and no society and few individuals in the region have been untouched by its influence. Throughout the PICs it is the most educated who migrate first, while many migrants have left rural areas to take advantage of superior urban and international educational facilities. These two factors in migration tend to reinforce each other so that this bias is likely to be maintained. Invariably, migration has resulted in the loss of the most energetic, skilled and innovative individuals, and this loss is not necessarily compensated either by remittances or by other trickle-down effects from urban and national development.

In some small states the brain drain has been excessive. Cook Islands, for example, lost more than half its vocationally qualified population in a decade, 1966-76, (Cook Islands, 1984:23) and much the same happened again in the mid-1990s when the national economy collapsed. In the case of migration of Tongans and Samoans to the United States of America, "Emigration results in the permanent loss of young educated skilled labour from the Pacific island countries. Skilled labour is in short supply and emigration probably hinders development" (Ahlburg and Levin, 1990: 84). This is certainly true more generally in the health sector where more costly (and sometimes less skilled) replacements have sometimes been required. It is widely true within the government sector in Samoa (Liki, 1994) and almost certainly evident elsewhere.

The ubiquity of the education bias in migration, despite the short history of formal education in some parts of the Pacific, suggests that the loss of skills is likely to continue. Indeed the fragmentary evidence that is available for the 1990s suggests that this has indeed continued, and that because of increased restrictions on immigration in metropolitan states, this bias has been, if anything, accentuated. Moreover skilled migrants are more easily and more likely to migrate following political or other problems, as was the case in Fiji in both 1987 and 2000. The combination of changing aspirations and the migration of educated young people contributes to the brain and skill drain from national peripheries and from small states, perhaps ultimately worsening the welfare and bargaining position of those places.

A few studies have been undertaken of return migration in the Pacific. The limited early evidence available suggested that "returnees" were mostly those who had retired or failed to secure employment or become successful. However that may disguise some degree of return migration of the relatively skilled (Liki, 2001) and, at the very least, return migration across a wide range of categories (Maron, 2001). However, the volume of return migration is small relative to the flow outwards. Despite stated intentions, "It is probably unrealistic to expect more than a tiny fraction of those who have already escaped ever to go back. Many will want to go back but only if this want is never put to the test" (Crocombe, 1978:2). In some cases return migration is perceived as an admission of failure.

The limited extent of return migration is at least in part due to the great differences in income levels between the PICs and the metropolitan periphery. It may also be a function of the general situation where the children of migrants are being educated in the destination country and, in some cases, may have lost some degree of contact with 'home' societies even to the extent where they have lost linguistic skills, and thus both parents and children would be embarrassed by the prospect, for example, of "young Samoans returning home unable to speak their own language" (Emery, 1976: 16). In turn this is also linked to a gradual shift in the demographic balance, especially from Polynesian states to the metropolitan fringe; relatives are increasingly likely to be found in destinations. Despite occasional pressures on migrants who live overseas and occasional incentives from within the Pacific, the volume of return migration is small.

In the context of migration from Samoa, it has been bluntly stated, "Polynesian migrants do not return except for visitations, once they are overseas and have attained a degree of security" (Shankman, 1976:96). On the other hand, overseas education and employment may bring return migrants both status and deference and high relative incomes at home (Marcus 1981:60). For Cook Islands, many skilled, qualified and experienced people have returned to the islands and been able to use their skills in a range of occupations, not merely in the public service (Hooker and Varcoe, 1999: 96), though Cook Islands is unusual in that wages and salaries in the islands are somewhat comparable with those in the principal destination, New Zealand. Nonetheless these studies suggest that there may be some selectivity towards the return migration of the relatively skilled or, at the very least, there is some potential for this, in appropriate circumstances.

A detailed analysis of attitudes to return migration among Samoans in New Zealand concluded that there were four principal reasons for non-return. First, local businesses succeeded only rarely, partly because commerce was poorly understood, and partly because social pressures from extended family eroded profitability (and, more recently, because available niches of opportunity have sometimes been hard to find); hence there was a reluctance to return to the private sector. Second, wages and fringe benefits in Samoa were very low. Third, New Zealand-born children had trouble adjusting to Samoa; hence parents were reluctant to return with them. Fourth, the gerontocratic social organization limited the scope for individual aspirations (Macpherson 1983). Overall, therefore, return migrants were unable, or felt they were unable, to return to a social context where they perceived that the rewards and opportunities for individual development were relatively limited. In this case, potential return migrants clearly addressed the notion of return primarily in terms of their entry into the private sector; hence their rationale may be inappropriate for potential return migrants to the public sector. However the role of both extended families and children born overseas is likely to be rather similar. Demographic factors are influential in return migration.

Almost every analysis of migration in the Pacific region points to the ways in which migration may be structured and analysed, but ultimately migration is often contingent on a complex variety of factors which defy easy categorization and make analysis of the rationale for migration (let alone policy formation) somewhat difficult. This is readily evident in the following abbreviated account of the migration history of a Cook Islands nurse.

> In 1965 Tevai was born in Aitutaki, one of the southern islands in the Cook Islands group. ... [After an unsettled year with relatives in Tahiti, her parents] decided that she should go to New Zealand to live with some other relatives. Tevai didn't settle to life in New Zealand at all, and after three months the family sent her to live with her older brother and his family. ... Tevai found a niche in Australia and after finishing high school went on to train as a nurse. Tevai had been working in Sydney as a nurse for six months when her father died and she was called back to her family in Aitutaki. The family asked Tevai if she would take over the responsibility of caring for her mother. Tevai agreed and for the next few years adopted a dual lifestyle, living alternatively in Aitutaki and Australia. In Australia Tevai earned good wages nursing and was able to send part of her wages home to her mother. While staying on Aitutaki she and her mother lived a fairly subsistence lifestyle. ... As her mother became ill, however, Tevai found it necessary to spend more and more time in Aitutaki. In 1991 she applied for a full-time nursing job at the hospital on Rarotonga. ... Tevai got the job. Although she considered her wage to be very poor compared with wages received in Australia, Tevai wanted to live closer to her mother. Recently, after her mother's sixtieth birthday, the family had a meeting and decided that Tevai had done her share of looking after her mother, and that Tevai's sister would come back from Australia to take over. Tevai wants to go back to Australia in a couple of years to earn some more but intends to return to Rarotonga eventually and build a house on the land given to her by her mother (quoted in Hooker and Varcoe, 1999: 95).

While this migration history is unusually complex, it is illustrative of the very real complexities of migration that do occur in the Pacific region, and, above all, the manner in which families and family responsibilities are linked to migration. In this context, as in others, it is evident that the structure of migration was in large part unrelated to considerations of skilled employment.

In some contexts in the region international migration has been viewed as a kind of 'safety valve', reducing pressures on national governments to provide employment opportunities and welfare services especially in conditions of high rates of natural increase of population and low rates of economic growth. Thus, at a national level in virtually all the sending countries of the region (except Niue), there is little general concern over the extent of international migration but only concerns related to specific issues, such as the 'brain drain' (or the developmental use of remittances). Throughout the region the 'safety valve' effect, limited economic growth plus concern over individual freedom of movement, have combined to result in steady and domestically unimpeded migration from many countries.

What is particularly critical in small PICs is that it is unusually difficult to replace skilled migrants, both because of the duration of training that is required and the very small demand for some particular skills. Thus a recent report on the health workforce in Tonga observed:

> With the resignation of one physiotherapist from the Physiotherapy Unit staff earlier this year, the unit is staffed by only one qualified physiotherapist. The remaining staff member...has been an employee of the Ministry for the past 18 years. The unit has been without a second physiotherapist for many months – the physiotherapist who had been studying overseas did not return to Tonga on completing her training... There is no likelihood of recruiting a Tongan national to fill the vacant physiotherapist post within the foreseeable future. Recruitment of a school-leaver to a newly created post of physiotherapy aide is required... The employment of this aide does not of course answer the need to train a second professional physiotherapist. It will be necessary to select a student to go to FSM [Fiji School of Medicine] to complete the physiotherapy diploma course there as soon as possible (Dewdney, 2000).

Not only could similar kinds of observations be recorded for other similarly specialized health positions, including pharmacy and radiology, but also for other PICs. Thus in Vanuatu, the principal skills that were missing in the two main urban hospitals were non-clinical skills, including planning and management, budget control, statistical analysis, and computer skills (Vanuatu Ministry of Health, 2000). In Tonga, it was evident not only that was there no immediate prospect of gaining a recruit to go to the Fiji School of Medicine (or even necessarily a school leaver aide); hence the "as soon as possible" was indefinite, but also that the whole procedure was utterly unpredictable. While this is less likely to be true for the nurses and doctors that are the focus of the present study, since numbers are rather larger, it is even truer in the smallest PICs. It is equally evident that, because of the necessity for appropriate skilled training, it is more difficult to substitute for (or transfer from elsewhere in the public service) absent skills in the health workforce.

Overall, the available evidence on international migration in the Pacific islands demonstrates that in the short-run a number of distinct benefits accrue to individual migrants and their families and to the sending societies. Despite rising unemployment and recession in destination countries, this appears to remain true. Migration has reduced the level of open and disguised unemployment, despite the loss of skilled human resources from the 'modern' sector, and reduced population pressure on scarce land resources at times. Migrant remittances have contributed to various facets of national and household development; they have raised living standards, contributed to employment (especially in the service and construction sectors) and eased balance of payments problems, despite contributing to inflation, especially in the larger Polynesian countries of Samoa and Tonga.

So substantial have these linkages been that, as in the case of Tonga, overseas migrants have been seen as simply one element of a 'transnational corporation of kin' (Marcus 1981). Such a structure, as seen elsewhere, may seek to maximize extended household incomes across different continents, and in doing so not only helps to maintain and enhance these family and communal networks but also provides the most substantial household rationale for overseas migration. There is no reason to believe that skilled migrants are any less part of such networks than unskilled migrants, especially since their earning power is substantially greater, while the notion of a 'transnational corporation of kin' now extends far beyond Tonga alone. Migration is therefore highly likely to be embedded in strategies for extended household development, rather than being the outcome of decisions taken by a very small number of individuals.

The significance of migration and the ensuing remittances has been such that the smaller island states (initially specifically Kiribati, Tokelau, Cook Islands and Tuvalu) have been conceptualized as states where migration, remittances, aid and the resultant largely urban bureaucracy are central to the socioeconomic system of those states (Bertram and Watters, 1985). While this image is disliked in the Pacific, because of its implication of a 'handout mentality', it nonetheless suggests the centrality of migration in PICs, and has been largely unchallenged for two decades (Bertram, 1999). Moreover it has been seen as an appropriate description of the situation in various other small PICs and elsewhere (Connell, 1988). In a very real sense therefore international migration has long had a critical and virtually uncontested role in island societies and economies. The migration of skilled workers thus needs to be seen in this broad context of continuity.

Long-term migration may impose considerable costs. Little of the income remitted was invested. Governments have not been able to control or direct the use of remittances (and nor have they generally sought to do so), while the rising material consumption levels following migration tend to generate increased demand for consumer goods. This demand, and other parallel demands for superior lifestyles, can usually only be met through further migration, as long as other forms of economic growth prove difficult to develop. Unfortunately there is every reason to believe this is unlikely to change in the immediate future and some reason to believe that the prospects for economic development in PICs are likely to worsen.

All the generalizations discussed above have been based on limited data from a few reliable but widely dispersed (in time and space) studies; hence many questions have not been thoroughly investigated. This is particularly true of studies of the migration of skilled individuals, and of return migration to the PICs. There are so few of these that all conclusions must be hedged with considerable caution and, indeed, despite exceptions, what is true of one island state (or even one island) may not be true of any other. For these reasons alone, and because of the particular role of skilled individuals in the region, a study of skilled migration has long been overdue.

2.2 ISLAND STATES AND THE HEALTH WORKFORCE

The Pacific island region, as conventionally defined, consists of some 22 states and almost a thousand language groups in an area of exceptional geographical, cultural and economic diversity, complicated by fragmentation, restricted land areas and the isolation of small islands and island states. Crudely the larger Melanesian states in the west have been characterized by internal migration, the Polynesian states to the east by extensive international migration and the smaller Micronesian states to the north by both internal and increasingly international migration. The most substantial emigration streams in the region have come from the central Polynesian states (Tonga, Samoa, Niue, Cook Islands and Tokelau), Fiji and, to a lesser extent, the Micronesian states of Palau, the Marshall Islands and the Federated States of Micronesia. With the exception of the very small and politically dependent Polynesian territories, and two of the Micronesian states, these states are the focus of this report.

The prospects for sustained economic development in PICs have generally been considered to be poor in comparison with many other regions of the world. There are now widely perceived differences in economic welfare between the PICs and those of the metropolitan fringe, and this has resulted in migration from the PICs to the Pacific periphery. In 1999-2000, some of the difficulties attached to social and economic development have been reflected in a series of political crises particularly within the Melanesian states. There is however considerable

Table 1. Pacific Populations

	Population	Population density (persons per sq km)	Population growth rate	Urban population (%)	Total fertility rate	Life expectancy at birth
FSM	118 100	168	1.9	30	4.9	65.7
Fiji	824 700	45	1.6	50	2.6	66.5
Kiribati	90 700	112	2.5	39	4.5	61.5
Marshall Islands	51 800	286	2.0	65	5.7	67.5
Palau	19 100	39	2.2	74	2.6	69.0
PNG	4 790 800	10	2.3	18	4.8	53.5
Samoa	169 200	58	0.6	24	4.5	68.4
Solomon Islands	447 900	16	2.8	18	5.7	61.4
Tonga	100 200	154	0.6	32	4.2	70.7
Tuvalu	9900	381	0.9	44	3.4	67.0
Vanuatu	199 800	16	3.0	22	5.3	64.2

Source: Secretariat of the Pacific Community, 2001

diversity within the PICs. Other than Papua New Guinea, Fiji is the only state with more than 500 000 people (having about 825 000) followed by Solomon Islands with 448 000 people. Vanuatu, Solomon Islands and the Marshall Islands are rapidly growing, through relatively high rates of natural increase, while some of the smaller states, including Tonga (with about 100 000 people) and Samoa (with about 170 000 people) have more or less static populations because of high rates of emigration. The Melanesian states in the south and western Pacific have low population densities, whereas Tonga and the atoll states have high densities. All of the PICs experience low or even negative rates of economic growth. Limited land areas, few natural resources, isolation and fragmentation, and weak infrastructures all pose problems for administration and development.

2.3 HEALTH

Health status varies considerably within the Pacific and is least adequate in the large Melanesian states and best in those states politically dependent on metropolitan nations (Taylor et al., 1991). Even between the independent PICs, there are considerable variations; thus life expectancies in Fiji and Tonga exceed that in Kiribati by several years (Table 1). These differences are partly a function of striking differences in economic and social development that reflect the isolated and more limited social development in the Melanesian states.

Countries are at various stages of the epidemiological transition, from a situation where the causes of morbidity and mortality are dominated by infection, acute respiratory disease and under-nutrition to one where noncommunicable diseases (especially cardiovascular disease, diabetes and cancer) and external causes (such as accidents) are the principal causes (Lewis and Rapaport, 1995). In recent years, there has been some re-emergence of infectious diseases, notably tuberculosis and yaws (in Melanesia), alongside the rapid growth of HIV/AIDS, not only in Melanesia, but also in Kiribati (Connell, 1997). The transition has been most evident in the Polynesian states and in more 'modern' areas elsewhere, and particularly the urban areas.

The epidemiological transition has been paralleled by a demographic transition from high birth and death rates to low birth and death rates. However, in most countries the transition is effectively incomplete and population growth remains rapid in several countries, especially Vanuatu, Solomon Islands and the Marshall Islands. Elsewhere, rapid population growth has been slowed, but largely by the 'safety valve' of international migration. Longer life expectancies, ageing and growing populations and the rise of noncommunicable diseases have placed increased stress on health care systems in the PICs.

Medical systems were introduced into most Pacific colonies in the nineteenth century, with hospitals usually being in the port towns and staffed by doctors and nurses from the missions or the colonial administration. Rural populations were relatively poorly served, and more often by missionary endeavour, though rural health clinics became more prevalent from the 1950s and were often staffed by local people. The relatively late arrival of medical services in several places has meant that traditional beliefs about the causes and cures of disease are common in several areas, and two models of health care persist (e.g. Hamnett and Connell, 1981; McGrath, 1999). Generally, however, dual and local systems have been replaced by a centralized hierarchical health system.

The modern health care system has tended to become more centralized, in its effectiveness, to the extent that in several states there are particular concerns about the delivery of health care services to remote and rural areas and, as in Papua New Guinea, a clear recognition that rural areas are inadequately served (Thomason et al., 1991). In this context at least mortality levels are actually increasing and life expectancies declining (Connell, 1997). In some PICs, improvements in life expectancy have slowed, or even reversed. This situation is linked to economic stagnation from the 1980s onwards which posed problems for achieving adequate nutritional outcomes, and meant that there were substantial reductions in real government spending on health (World Bank, 1994). Thus in Vanuatu the number of village health workers declined by two thirds between 1991 and 1992 with the collapse of financial support for their activities (op cit: 279). Similar reconstructions occurred elsewhere to the detriment of remote areas.

Primary health care has been widely advocated, in terms of a more equitable distribution of more appropriate resources and a greater focus on environmental health, while the more specific notion of 'Healthy Islands' has also been advocated, with the Fijian island of Kadavu as the prototype (Han, 1996). However, new directions have been hampered by weak political commitment, a dependence on historic models (sometimes engendered by the constraints of aid delivery) including the construction and maintenance of central hospitals, and a lack of vision. Indeed it has been argued:

Governments are building hospitals, attracting more technology, increasing medical specialization, and minimally reorienting the medical curriculums for doctors and nurses, while often neglecting the needs of rural people [while] physicians and other health professionals are worried that primary health care will decrease their income, status and influence. A common claim is that the quality of service will be threatened; but this can be a subterfuge. Health professionals generally have a disproportionate ownership of and access to both wealth and power and are in the self-gratifying position of being consumers of public funds and controllers of the health market (Pollock and Finau, 1999: 291).

All of this, alongside a relative and absolute lack of resources, has slowed the pace of change and emphasized the focus on hospital-based curative care (with resultant questions over equity) in Pacific health care systems.

In most PICs, the private health sector has hitherto been largely conspicuous by its absence, but it is now growing more rapidly. Previously, small populations (even in urban areas) a lack of means to pay and competition from the public sector (where most services have been virtually free) have meant that few private practitioners could be supported in the island states. Some large corporations, such as mining companies in Papua New Guinea, have brought in their own private medical care systems and sometimes extended those to local populations not directly involved in mining, but the emergence of a small private sector has followed frustrations with the public sector on the part of a small local elite. In Fiji, the private sector grew rapidly in the wake of the 1987 coups, as Fiji-Indians left the public sector, but this is exceptional. Elsewhere, though the private sector is small, as in the case of Samoa, it has resulted in a movement of workers from the public sector because of substantially different wage rates, into a sector that supports a very small proportion of the total population, and in several cases, again as in Samoa, that proportion is dominated by expatriates.

The organization of health administration is necessarily hierarchical but this is emphasized by a degree of authoritarianism which is not unusual in the region; this may also interact with authoritarian and centralized administrative structures that have been inherited from colonial times to produce what has been described as a "militaristic and inflexible bureaucracy" (Taylor, 1990: 105; cf. Finau, 1988). Such bureaucracies may appear, and sometimes are, autocratic to those in subordinate positions. The combination of hierarchy, authoritarianism and some degree of autocracy, in health care systems where the opportunities for promotion may be few, simply because there are few higher level positions, may be very frustrating for those at lower levels in the hierarchy. Indeed "the criteria for promotion or demotion become largely unrelated to technical ability, qualification or organizational needs" (Finau, 1988: 140). This may be a factor encouraging emigration, and it has certainly been indicated to be a more general factor in migration, especially from the Polynesian states (Shore, 1978), as opportunities for advancement are few.

Such bureaucratic systems are also poorly equipped to deal with the flexible specialization required in small island states. Conversely the small size of the bureaucracy emphasizes personal relationships. Taylor has observed, "In fact they live and work closely together for most of their lives. This makes many aspects of administration easier since each is familiar with the strengths and weaknesses of the other. The existing personal relationships through the health department often assist with the promotion of a sense of teamwork" (1990: 107). However, such intimate personal and professional relationships may not always be so harmonious, and tensions in the senior levels of bureaucracy are not unusual especially where there exist so few possibilities for change and restructuring. In certain circumstances there may even be a "power struggle between the professional staff, who are directly involved in the productive process, and the management who become overly concerned with internal efficiency" (Finau, 1988: 13). In such contexts, the goals of achievement of holistic health are lost in personalized bureaucratic structures.

Pacific health care systems vary considerably. Population per hospital bed ranges from under 50 to over 300 (in Fiji and the Solomon Islands, respectively), while the number of people per doctor ranges from under 1000 (in dependent territories) to over 15 000 in Papua New Guinea (Taylor, 1990; WHO, 1999). In all cases where information is available, only a small proportion of health budgets are allocated to primary health care. Similarly, the limited data available suggest an urban bias in health expenditure and personnel distribution, though this is unsurprising in the Pacific where the headquarters of the health department and the main referral (or only significant) hospital are located in the capital city, which is sometimes the only town (Taylor 1990). Hence access to health care and the quality of services are usually least adequate, and often inadequate, in remote areas. This deficiency, at least in terms of the distribution of personnel, has been documented in the case of Vanuatu where the two main hospitals were relatively well supplied with staff, the provincial hospitals lacked many skills (including emergency nursing skills, physiotherapy and rehabilitation skills) and the provincial health centres "demonstrated a dramatic increase in clinical and treatment skills gaps" (Vanuatu Ministry of Health, 2000). Such a situation is likely to be common elsewhere.

One outcome of a centralized and hierarchical medical care system is that central authorities tend to monopolize planning, budgeting and human resource recruitment and allocation functions. At the same time they may be reluctant to devolve some specific functions to the peripheral and outlying areas. Skilled health workers in most PICs have thus been reluctant to move to outlying areas, where there is little support for them from the line ministry and where other facilities may be exceptionally limited.

There is often a lack of material resources for health care in the PICs; this may include buildings, but is particularly true of supplies. Maintenance of expensive and complicated equipment is also a common problem, adding to the difficulties of providing adequate health care, and adding to the frustrations of those employed to achieve this. In most contexts, this is compounded by deficiencies at middle and peripheral levels in the health workforce, especially where there is a "tradition of moving the most competent administrators or people with quantitative/computer expertise to more 'important' sectors, such as economic statistics" (Taylor, 1990: 94). That situation has not subsequently changed.

The smallness of island populations means that specialization is not cost effective, in clinical, administrative and public health areas. In some PICs there is no clinical specialization at all, and in the larger countries there is some specialization into medicine, surgery, paediatrics etc. at the national level. Many directors of health, or even ministers, as in Tonga, may divide their time between bureaucratic management, the practice of general medicine and the performance of specialized surgical procedures. Specialization in areas of health administration is equally difficult; few if any island states have trained epidemiologists or health economists.

Because of small populations, self-sufficiency in medical and health resources at a level to which many aspire is simply not possible, even with reasonably high standards of living. 'Training highly specialized clinical, administrative and public health personnel is not only an inappropriate use of resources in the less-developed island countries with small populations, it is inappropriate no matter what the level of development" (Taylor, 1990: 90), since there is simply inadequate specialized work for some individuals. In some circumstances this may be a disincentive for those who have, or aspire to have, particular specializations, to remain in the health care system. It also means that where there are very few individuals with particular expertise, whether medical or administrative, their loss to the health system, because of emigration (or any other reason), is a greater loss to small island health care systems than within larger states.

One of the implications of limited specialization, lack of technology and specialized support services, and the absence (perhaps because of migration) of key individuals is that international referral and evacuation of medical cases is relatively common. However, this is especially true of those territories that remain politically dependent on metropolitan states where, at least in the American territories, it has become a 'costly and complex business'. In some PICs there exists a high level of expectation that people will be evacuated for diagnosis and treatment. During the early 1980s, the Marshall Islands spent about half its health budget on off-island referrals, mainly to Hawaii, and the figure in American Samoa was about one third (Taylor, 1990: 99). Attempts to reduce the referral rate have followed, but referrals remain an expensive issue, while simultaneously emphasizing the difficulties of achieving or retaining an adequate supply of health practitioners and facilities in small PICs.

As long as high levels of referrals continue, the health systems of PICs are likely to be regarded as inferior by many of the local population. Correspondingly, as long as there is a shortage of SHPs, referrals are more likely to occur (at some cost) for preventable conditions. This problem has been effectively summarized by the World Bank for the case of Samoa: "The problem of thin labor markets and the nature of the chronic and persistent supply-demand imbalances for specific skills need to be explicitly recognized and the problems addressed directly in planning for the health sector where many high level skills in small numbers are required to support health service delivery efforts" (1994: 324). Solutions to this problem, true of other sectors in small states, have not been easy to find.

Problems exist in the organization of local training of health personnel in small states. There are several nursing schools. However, training medical practitioners poses greater difficulties, even though there are two institutions for training in the Pacific: the University of Papua New Guinea (UPNG) in Port Moresby and the Fiji School of Medicine in Suva. For more than a decade, from the mid-1980s, there was also the Pacific Basin Medical Officers Training Program in Pohnpei (the Federated States of Micronesia), but it was closed in 1996. Many Pacific islanders had problems passing courses and attrition rates were high; hence there was some movement towards problem-based learning in both Suva and Ponhpei (Dever, Finau and Hunton, 1997). A number of islanders have gained access to medical schools in Australia, New Zealand and the United States of America, and, at least a decade ago, it was possible to conclude: "Sophisticated medical training such as this is often inappropriate since the technology on which it is based is not available in many Pacific island countries, and graduates of these medical schools have a particularly high non-return rate" (Taylor, 1990: 91). There is some evidence that this remains the case, despite the development of courses within the region, as doctors especially continue to be trained overseas.

Most PICs have nursing schools, but it has been argued that low secondary education standards may prove to be barriers to entry or completion of the course, and that many rural recruits come to the urban centre for training and then marry, never to return to the rural area (Taylor, 1990: 91). Similarly, it has been argued that "it may be necessary to find jobs in the health department (such as maintenance) for husbands of nurses in order that they will return to the rural setting" (ibid), a clear indication of the significance of family factors in employment and migration and of the difficulty in maintaining adequate health care systems in rural areas.

Training of paramedical workers such as radiographers, physiotherapists and laboratory technicians also poses difficulties since relatively few such workers are needed. Therefore, courses can only be run intermittently, or all such workers must be trained overseas. "Some small countries may require only one or two of a certain type of personnel, but if one migrates or dies unexpectedly the workforce is decimated" (Taylor, 1990: 91). Indeed, the migration of such specialized personnel is almost certainly a more acute problem for some PICs than the loss of doctors and nurses simply because numbers are so few and replacement is very difficult.

Postgraduate specialized medical training was entirely undertaken in metropolitan states until the end of the 1980s. "It often required many years, was accompanied by high levels of failure and also high non-return rates among the few who were successful" (Taylor, 1990: 92). Taylor consequently identified mechanisms for minimizing the excessive migration of health professionals from island states: "Local training in the home country, or other Pacific island countries, is one of the answers, and local Master degrees for specialist qualifications is one of the answers" (ibid). Since then, there has been little positive change, and staff losses at the Fiji School of Medicine have made it more difficult to offer specialist courses there.

The reductions in spending on health care systems in the Pacific that became evident in the 1980s and have subsequently continued have had a damaging result in sustaining a skilled health labour force. This is partly because the health delivery system in the PICs requires high and unvarying levels of skilled labour inputs to staff hospital-based curative activities, to operate peripheral facilities and to undertake various preventative services. Indeed, the World Bank concluded in the mid-1990s that one of the two distinctive features of what they identified as, the Pacific health paradigm was "its vulnerability to worker and/or skill shortages" (World Bank, 1994: 19). Thus, Fiji had high personnel vacancy rates averaging 9% of approved posts in the mid-1980s, while in 1987-88, deteriorating pay prospects and ethnic tensions led to the resignation of over 100 doctors including many senior specialists, most of whom later emigrated—a blow from which the health care system never recovered. Indeed, by 1989, the overall vacancy rate had risen to 14%.

The situation in Fiji is unique in the Pacific region in that two military coups in 1987 deposed the elected government in moves that were construed by many as opposition to the growing political role of the Fiji-Indian population. This prompted a political, economic and social crisis and very substantial emigration, not only of Fiji-Indians but other races as well. The loss of 100 doctors in a period of 12 months compared with the loss of 67 in the previous five years was an exceptional circumstance and had serious implications:

> This in itself has put a tremendous strain on the remaining doctors and on the health system as a whole. There has been some help in the form of doctors from China and Australia ... but unfortunately it will take many years to recover the lost expertise and personnel. An indirect result of the loss of doctors has been the inability of doctors in Fiji to go overseas for further study. Hence we cannot expect many doctors to gain postgraduate qualifications in the next few years. Many of the doctors who have left were young people who had returned to Fiji in the last eight years because they could see some real challenges for bettering the standard of medicine here. This represents a real loss. Similarly a substantial number of nurses and other medical support staff have been lost to Fiji. In private practice, too, some doctors have migrated, leaving many people without a family doctor (Mitchell, 1988: 77).

As this account indicates, in this case at least, it was not just the substantial loss of a large number of doctors and other medical workers but the fact that those who went may well have been the more competent and dedicated staff.

The pattern of high vacancy rates is repeated in other PICs. While Fiji relied on donor support and direct recruitment to compensate for the loss of health workers—with some 36 expatriate doctors being made available through the United Nations Volunteers programme in the most critical post-coup period. Other countries have resorted to other means. Samoa and Kiribati have kept many doctors in service past retirement age, and have also turned to expatriates (mainly United Nations Volunteers) who account for a third of the public sector (World Bank, 1994: 19). A similar reliance on expatriates is also extremely important in Palau, Vanuatu, Solomon Islands and the Marshall Islands.

Reliance on expatriates imposes certain costs, in terms of recruitment fees and some local expenses, while there are opportunity costs to the donor funds that support the expatriates. Hence Kiribati, at the start of the 1990s, had to rely on a doctor work force a quarter smaller than that in place a decade earlier. Moreover, there are other disadvantages: 'These individuals, who come from varied medical backgrounds and bring differing approaches and quality standards, often cannot speak the local language and can be difficult to integrate into ongoing service delivery (and training) routines" (World Bank, 1994: 19). In Kiribati, the local people believe that western-trained doctors are too impersonal and too busy, mainly because they are not emotionally involved with their patient.

> The foreign practitioners do not speak Gilbertese and need a translator. The interaction becomes too complicated and too impersonal, the patient feels insecure, uneasy and becomes too resentful towards the medical practitioner. This resentfulness is ... commonly expressed in the attitude of the patient to prescribe drugs, in that patients fail to take the prescribed medication (Chritensen, 1995: 103).

In the case of Samoa, overseas doctors "come from a diverse range of locations (e.g. India and Myanmar) trained in different traditions and often lacking appropriate language skills. This has a significant influence on their ability to train counterparts and in some cases to treat patients adequately" (op cit: 322). This may also affect migration within the Pacific region.

Other countries have sought different solutions to the loss of doctors. Tonga has developed a new category of Health Officer, trained in a limited two-year course within Tonga, and who largely runs rural health centres or works in hospital outpatient wards. Replacement of doctors in this way in Tonga, and also in Kiribati, has not been without controversy: "Public perceptions of their competence have been less than fully favorable" and there has been greater pressure on nurses and on the recruitment of nurses with superior skills" (World Bank, 1994: 322). In both Fiji and Samoa there has been a policy of employing retired local medical officers on a yearly contract basis to fill vacancies. In Samoa, too, the doctor shortage has led to a growing role for nurses. This loss has inhibited the performance of the health care system (especially in more remote areas) and the loss of doctors has placed greater pressure on nurses.

Irrespective of the value of expatriate doctors and other health professionals, there is always considerable expense (in time and money) attached to their recruitment, including sometimes long delays, the difficulty of finding the right recruit, the cost of recruitment and so on. This puts considerable pressures on bureaucracies who are sometimes poorly equipped to cope.

2.4 THE HUMAN RESOURCE CONTEXT

A basis for this study has been the quantification of the existing health workforce in the PICs, to determine where there are shortfalls in SHPS, and where this has recently changed, i.e. to develop an immediate appreciation of the extent to which supply problems are particularly acute in some states (at a national or regional level). In some other contexts, where there has been a substantial emigration of SHPs, as in India (and perhaps in the Philippines), there has been some argument that this does not constitute a brain or skill-drain, but that it may actually be an overflow (Oommen, 1989) in the sense that national needs are presently satisfied. It will be necessary to examine if this is the situation in any of the PICs, though available evidence suggests that it is extremely unlikely.

Studies of the migration of SHPs have made various observations concerning the effect of migration on health care, though there is often little solid empirical data to support these observations. They include:

(1) the loss of health skills (on the assumption that lost skills must necessarily result in worsened health care outcomes), especially in rural and remote areas;

(2) the reduced morale and greater workload of those SHPs who remain;

(3) the immigration of replacement SHPs (who may not have appropriate qualifications, or may lack the language, cultural sensitivity, etc. to deal with local issues); and

(4) the cost of referrals (both domestically and internationally) where local expertise is unavailable.

Overall, these suggest that health services have experienced reduced efficiency (e.g. delays in receiving acute emergency care and long waiting times for scheduled services), have become more costly and, perhaps, have experienced some reduction in equity of access.

None of the above-mentioned perceived effects of migration on health care have been examined closely or systematically, and there may be compensating tendencies (e.g. the aid-financed delivery of specialized heart and opthalmological services in some PICs), though these cannot be depended on to provide continuity, and do not contribute to long-term sustainable health care.

The last detailed overview of the health workforce stock in the PICs was undertaken in 1990 (Rotem and Dewdney, 1991), covering 12 PICs. It excluded some of those (e.g. the Marshall Islands, Niue and Tuvalu) where SHP migration is perceived to be a problem, though more summary data exist for subsequent years (WHO, 1999). The 1990 overview showed that there were already problems relating to the retention of SHPs in several states (e.g. the Federated States of Micronesia, Fiji, Palau, Tonga and Samoa), alongside shortages of skilled workers in certain areas. The study also noted that both Fiji and Samoa referred specifically to a 'brain drain', while both Palau and Samoa recorded high attrition rates for overseas trained health workers (few of whom returned). Since migration was not the particular focus of the study and information was not collected in a systematic or consistent manner, the deficiencies that were reported were certainly only a fraction of those that existed. Moreover, since then, migration has evidently accelerated and has been particularly problematic in the smaller states, such as Kiribati and Tuvalu, both in numbers and in the proportion of the skilled health workforce that this represents.

The study sought to examine data on the stock (and shortfalls) of all categories of SHPs in the PICs; however, owing to the very different classifications that have been used, and doubts about the reliability of data, this was not as valuable as anticipated. It is, however, evident that there are relatively few doctors, and low doctor-patient ratios in the smaller island states (especially Kiribati, Tuvalu and Palau). In states with continued political relationships with metropolitan powers, such as Guam, the Northern Mariana Islands and New Caledonia, the situation was the reverse because of superior wages and facilities. For the states that were central to this study – Fiji, Samoa, Tonga and Vanuatu – the situation had changed relatively little in the 1990s. Fiji and Vanuatu both experienced a worsening of doctor-patient and nurse-patient ratios, whereas in Tonga and Samoa there had been some improvement in ratios. More generally in the region, where the numbers of doctors, nurses and other medical personnel had increased, that increase was at much the same rate or less than that of the population growth. Other than in those states that were linked to metropolitan powers, there was no significant improvement in the availability of SHPs in the 1990s.

Governments in the Pacific have attempted to determine the most appropriate models to provide comprehensive primary health care services to rural, remote and sparsely populated areas, atolls and outer islands. One issue is a shortage of doctors in most PICs. Of necessity, the few doctors in the workforce tend to be concentrated in referral hospitals in the main population centres. But even if there were more doctors, it would not be cost-effective to deploy these highly trained health workers in remote rural areas because the populations are so small and the health facilities in these communities have limited diagnostic and therapeutic equipment and supplies. Yet, because referral and transport of the sick and injured from these areas can be so difficult and can take long, the health workers posted to these small communities need excellent skills. This is why many countries have trained mid-level practitioners (MLPs). Each country's unique geography, socioeconomic structure, population size, distribution and health needs have influenced the role development of the heath care workers or MLPs who provide primary health care services in these remote areas.

MLPs are front-line health workers in the community. They are not doctors, but they have been trained to diagnose and treat common health problems, to manage emergencies, to refer appropriately and to transfer the seriously ill or injured for further care. Throughout the PICs, most MLPs have the same function – the provision of clinical primary health care in community-based health facilities. However, MLP education programmes vary considerably, as do the seriousness and complexity of health problems they can manage. Graduates of MLP courses have been given various titles, such as physician assistant, medex, medical assistant, health assistant and health officer. Nurses who undertake this advanced training are often called nurse practitioners. These titles do not always reflect the entry requirements or the level of training. Some MLPs with equivalent training are given different titles in different countries. For example, the role and training of nurse aids in Solomon Islands and community health workers in Papua New Guinea are similar. At the same time, some MLPs with different educational backgrounds may have similar titles. A medical assistant in Kiribati is a nurse who has received advanced training. A medical assistant in Fiji does not have a nursing background. Even MLPs with similar educational backgrounds and training have different titles in different countries. For example, medical assistants in Fiji, health officers in Tonga and health extension officers in Papua New Guinea are basically equivalent in their role, training and function.

Regardless of titles, MLPs have played an important role in meeting the health care needs (both preventive and curative) of the PICs, especially in remote or rural areas and sparsely populated locations where it is not cost effective to post a doctor. These health professionals play vital roles in meeting the needs of at-risk and vulnerable communities, including the poor, chronically ill, young and elderly.

WHO has supported the training of medical assistants in Kiribati; health assistants in the Marshall Islands and the Federated States of Micronesia; nurse practitioners in Cook Islands, Samoa and Vanuatu; and health officers in Tonga. Support has also been provided for the training of rural health workers (nurse aids) in Solomon Islands. Most recently, in September 1998, WHO cooperated in the development and evaluation of a new nurse practitioner programme in Fiji. The role and function of MLPs in the health workforce has been discussed for the past six years in WHO meetings of ministers of health of PICs. At the March 1999 meeting in Palau, the ministers of health requested WHO to undertake an assessment study of MLPs in the Pacific and to report the findings.

3

STUDY RATIONALE AND METHODOLOGY

For more than a quarter of a century, attention has been given to the gradual rise in the volume of skilled migration globally and the manner in which this constitutes a growing proportion of all international migration, as movement of unskilled workers and family members becomes more difficult. The rise in migration of skilled workers has been perceived as a response to the accelerated globalization of industrialization and the expansion and internationalization of the service sector. While the latter has primarily been seen in terms of financial services, it has long been evident that such professional services as health care are very much part of the new internationalization of labour.

A more recent dimension of international skilled migration has been the movement of students, whose numbers are now substantial and appear to be increasing. Moreover, the international movement of students "represents the internationalization of knowledge, and is arguably the most effective vehicle for creating a global migratory elite" (Koser and Salt, 1997). It therefore has the potential to be a critical, and pump-priming part of a substantial subsequent brain drain.

Much of the literature on international migration has focused on the notion of a brain and skill drain (e.g. Findlay, 1991; de Wenden, 1995) and involves three elements: first, the loss of productive skilled labour from countries where it is, or could be, potentially useful; second, the extent to which such losses are compensated by the return migration of individuals with superior skills (following training or employment experience overseas) or by flows of remittances; and third, the manner in which skilled migrants may be underutilized in destinations to the extent that migration results in skill loss rather than a brain gain.

The few previous studies of the movement of SHPs in the region have focused almost entirely on the out-migration of SHPs from the PICs (and, to a very much lesser extent, on the migration of SHPs into cities) and have not examined either the migration of Pacific island SHPs within the region, or the in-migration of SHPs from outside the region (mainly from Asia). The available evidence suggests that the last of these is of growing importance and necessitates careful examination.

The migration of SHPs is no new phenomenon. At least as early as 1989, a medical degree from the Fiji School of Medicine was regarded by some as a 'passport to prosperity'. However, there have been virtually no studies of 'movers': the out-migration of SHPs (and even fewer of other skilled migrants, where there is good reason to believe that parallels exist). The few studies that do exist focus primarily on individual aspirations, and only secondarily on doctors and nurses (Naidu, 1997; Rotem and Bailey, 1999). A recent study undertaken for the Commonwealth Secretariat (Rotem and Bailey, 1999) provided an overview of the situation in nine PICs but excluded some (such as the Federated States of Micronesia) where mobility is perceived to be a problem. Naidu (1997) considered only Fiji. The few studies that exist of the migration of SHPs in other parts of the world, such as that on doctors moving from Canada to the United States of America (McKendry et al., 1996), of nurses moving from the Philippines (Ishi, 1987; Ball, 1996) and of the internal mobility of female doctors within Mexico (Harrison, 1998), appear to be of limited relevance to the situation in the PICs, being in either rich world countries and/or in contexts with very different stock situations. In short, there are surprisingly few good studies in the Pacific or elsewhere of the migration of SHPs.

Existing studies of the PICs emphasize that migration is primarily related to quality of life issues that involve the particular employment context (poor working conditions, inadequate facilities, limited opportunities for research or career development), income (particular professional salary structures, costs of living) and a variety of social factors (educational opportunities for children, morale), though not necessarily in that order. A similar range of factors is usually assumed to also account for the migration of SHPs to capital cities in the region and to take up employment with regional institutions. None of these factors are surprising; they parallel similar conclusions elsewhere, but they do not necessarily provide a sophisticated understanding of migration. First, they focus on 'acceptable' explanations (those that make immediate sense to interviewer and interviewee) but have little to say about wider family and social obligations (such as the expectations of others, including graduating cohorts), personal 'politics' (culture and hierarchy in the health context and in the wider society), which may be of considerable importance. Second, they say nothing about some variables that might be expected to be of particular significance, including gender and marital status. Third, they are not linked to an institutional context, in the sense that individual orientations are historically shaped in a training and work environment, and in a social context, which develop and provide certain expectations.

With one partial exception, there appear to have been no studies of why SHPs (or other skilled workers) remain in the PICs. That exception, a study of a group of doctors in Fiji, indicated that the two most significant, yet vague, factors for 'stayers' remaining were "job satisfaction" and "lifestyle" (Naidu, 1997: 70-71). However, what these actually constituted and whom they most influenced were not recorded (although there is some evidence that they were not necessarily older individuals). It may also be that the particular balance between public and private sector employment (and the wages and salaries in the two sectors) is of considerable importance. Clearly, it is extremely important to ascertain what factors do influence the retention of health personnel.

Equally important, there has also been some return migration of skilled workers from overseas; this has never been effectively studied in the health sector, and there has been virtually no examination of return migration in the PICs, probably primarily because of the assumption that this is rare. Again, it is critically important to examine where and why this has occurred, and hence what prospects and policies exist for attracting more return migration of SHPs.

There have been no studies of the migration of SHPs into the PICs (and no good studies of other skilled immigrants into the PICs), since this is a rather more difficult undertaking. However it is necessary to undertake such a study to establish the role and qualifications of immigrant SHPs - the 'arrivals' - in the region, the anticipated duration of their stay and their impact on health care in the region. The minimal evidence that exists suggests that SHP 'arrivals' are most evident in the Compact states of Micronesia (Palau, the Federated States of Micronesia, and the Marshall Islands) and also in some parts of Melanesia (from Papua New Guinea to Fiji).

The core of this study is a series of surveys of SHP movers, stayers and arrivals, which will focus on doctors (medical officers) and graduate nurses, partly to build on the few previous studies, and partly because their numbers (whether movers, stayers or arrivals) appear to be greater than those in any other category. This is not to suggest that the impact of the loss of individuals in other categories (e.g. medical specialists, radiographers) is not equally or even more severe (where it may result in costly referrals or undiagnosed conditions or both), but their numbers only justify a specific survey when the impact of emigration is considerable.

The two most favoured destinations for movers outside the region appear to be Australia (Sydney) and New Zealand (Auckland), though there may be a growing number of SHPs in the United States of America, especially in Hawaii. Though there are some reasons why the migration of SHPs to the United States of America is likely to be different from that in the southern hemisphere (e.g. migration from Micronesia, more privatized health care) the study focused on the two destinations of Sydney and Auckland, and on three key migrant groups: Tongans, Samoans and Fijians (including Fiji-Indians). As far as possible, data were collected for smaller groups, including those from Cook Islands, Niue and Tokelau (whose numbers overseas are quite small but the consequence of whose migration can be considerable). A smaller study was undertaken of Fiji-Indian migrants in Vancouver, Canada. The studies focused on household structure, training, the rationale for migration, careers (the labour market experience) and the potential for future stability or migration (including return migration) of present migrant SHPs (see Appendix 1: Questionnaires). Samples were developed in conjunction with the migrant communities, academic researchers and medical organizations, and include both those who have remained employed in the health sector and those who have left (although the difficulties in tracing the latter group have meant that there were very few of them).

Within the PICs, parallel surveys of local nurses and doctors were undertaken in the key countries of origin (Tonga, Samoa and Fiji, and also in Vanuatu and Palau) and focused on similar themes alongside attitudes to the health profession and the propensity to migrate. These were entirely undertaken in the capital cities because of logistical and economic considerations, hence excluding other centres (where pressures on SHPs, and the propensity to migrate, may be somewhat greater, and demand for adequate health care less likely to be satisfied).

The final core element of study focused on the immigration of doctors and nurses into the PICS; this concentrated on Fiji, Palau and Vanuatu, where numbers were relatively high. A brief but somewhat inconclusive survey was also undertaken of SHPs currently in training in Sydney.

The aim was to undertake a core study of about 150 'movers', mainly in the two destination countries (approximately half each in Australia and New Zealand); a similar number of 'stayers' (about 50 in Fiji and 25 each in Tonga, Samoa, Vanuatu and Palau); and, a rather smaller number of 'arrivals' (about 25 in Fiji and about 20 each in the Federated States of Micronesia, Samoa, Tonga and Vanuatu). These studies were undertaken by experienced research assistants who had, as far as possible, some links with the relevant communities. For a variety of reasons, it proved extremely difficult to undertake studies in certain countries at certain times and especially in the metropolitan countries; hence the number of migrants was fewer than anticipated. Nonetheless, over 280 questionnaires were completed.

The complexity of international migration is considerable. Economic variables, and especially the relationship between income levels and cost of living, are generally considered to be of key relevance in influencing migration decisions. According to human capital theory, people tend to migrate if predicted earnings (estimated relevant to age, education and years of work experience) and real incomes set against costs of living are greater in the place (or country) of destination. While this was expected to be of some importance in the proposed study, it was also expected that in the context of both 'movers' and, to a lesser extent, 'stayers', social variables would also prove to be of considerable significance. Migration now has a substantial history in the region, overseas social networks (the 'transnational corporation of kin') are extensive, access to education for family members is important and social status is of some concern in much of the region. All of this is tied into the conditions and location of training facilities. Taylor simply concluded that for PICs, "Migration is more likely if an individual had recognisable qualifications in the destination country, lived there for some period, and particularly if married to a national of that country – all are often a consequence of overseas professional training" (1990: 92). The balance between such variables and many others is likely to vary significantly between places and social categories.

The following sections examine in detail these kinds of explanations and correlations in the context of the surveys undertaken in the region during the recent study period, alongside other available information. In every case, the results and conclusions must be regarded as preliminary, while it is not yet possible to compare the results of surveys within countries with those outside the countries. Hence the most important element of the analysis – the comparison of movers and stayers – is yet to be undertaken.

4
FINDINGS

4.1 FIJI

Other than Papua New Guinea, Fiji is by far the largest island state in the Pacific region, with a population of around 840 000, and with a more complex economy than any other. The economy is heavily dependent on sugar and tourism. The former was experiencing problems even before the 2000 coup, which severely affected both key elements of the economy, while also devastating the largest industrial economy in the Pacific region. The economy has yet to recover from these crises.

Fiji also has the largest, most complex and developed health care system in the Pacific region. It also has the health care system that has been most affected by emigration, especially in the last 15 years, when ethnic tensions and military coups have prompted a series of resignations and departures, notably after the coups in 1987 and 2000. After 1987, private health services also increased significantly, with attrition from the public sector.

A shortage of doctors first became evident in the country around 1977 when a number of local medical graduates resigned to run their own private medical clinics. Prior to that, graduates of the Fiji School of Medicine (FSM) were not allowed to practise in the private sector. Fiji has 18 hospitals and nearly 3000 employees in the health care system, while there is also a substantial and growing private health care system. Until 1987, the availability of adequate skilled human resources was not a problem in Fiji. Now it is, although even the very substantial loss of personnel in the last 13 years may still not have made the labour supply problem as difficult as in other parts of Melanesia.

After the 1987 coups, the health service deteriorated, partly because of the loss of skilled labour and the economic decline, which reduced capital availability for development. There was a widespread feeling that public concerns over declining standards were being ignored, at least partly because the Ministry was unable to easily resolve them. A senior official of the Fiji Medical Association, for example, stated that a crisis looms in "our hospitals and the Government does not seem to want to address it" and added that "the shortage of adequately skilled and experienced doctors was affecting the quality of care" (*Fiji Times*, 30 September 1995, quoted by Naidu, 1997: 4). It was also argued that one of the secondary consequences of the coup was that new vacancies at senior levels in the public sector were being filled by under-qualified applicants on the basis of ethnicity rather than ability (ibid).

> At much the same time, Prime Minister Sitiveni Rabuka maintained:
>
> The emigration of doctors is a drain on Fiji's professional and human resource. Some say the reason they left the country is political. This is an easy excuse that is really a rationalization of the real reasons for emigration, and that is the wider opportunities for a more comfortable life overseas. I believe doctors who were born here should show more dedication to Fiji and make their contribution to their people, rather than going off to sell their services to richer people in those countries (*Fiji Times*, 13 May 1966, quoted in Naidu, 1997: 31).

Such appeals to altruism had no effect in a context where changes to the health system, or to the wider national context, were missing. Indeed, such appeals to a dominantly Fiji-Indian medical profession were construed as an unwillingness to deal with more complex issues.

Parallel changes were going on in other parts of the health sector, although these were less easy to demonstrate because of the small numbers in particular categories. The number of dentists fell from 67 in 1986, to 48 by the end of 1987 and to 40 in 1994 (Gani, 1999: 99). In dentistry, the majority of the skilled professionals were Fiji-Indians.

In the late 1990s, there remained a shortage of doctors and considerable work pressure was put on those in place. In 1996, there were 145 expatriate doctors and 62 vacancies in a total establishment of 383 doctors. It was said that all ward doctors were expected to be on call for two nights a week, with $1 per night remuneration, and "were constantly looking for alternative employment" out of concern that not enough was being done by the government to remedy the deficit (Naidu, 1997: 60). Between 1984 and 1994, Fiji lost 586 doctors through emigration (although proportionately the decline was less than it was for teachers). The loss of SHPs was part of a much larger emigration of skilled workers.

According to a survey undertaken in 1996, the mean age of emigrant doctors was 34 compared with the mean age of a sample of doctors within Fiji of 42. Younger doctors, presumably the more skilled, were thus the most likely to have migrated (Naidu, 1997: 66). Overseas trained doctors were more likely to have emigrated than those trained within Fiji (op cit: 67), although, as elsewhere, that distinction may have been already present in the choice of training location. There was a significant difference between those doctors resident in Fiji who were employed in the public and private sectors, in that those in the private sector enjoyed more job satisfaction and greater monetary rewards.

The study undertaken in 1997 by Naidu revealed that the most frequently cited reason given by more than a third of all doctors who had already migrated was the poor working conditions in Fiji's public hospitals. This was followed in descending order of significance by political instability, low salary, inadequate facilities, and, finally, the limited scope for postgraduate medical training in Fiji for those who wished to pursue a specialization. In combination, these had contributed to low morale (Naidu, 1997: 67). Some doctors perceived the root cause of their emigration to lie in the low calibre of the administrative personnel in the headquarters of the Ministry of Health. One observed that "the Ministry of Health, its Ministers, the Permanent Secretary and most of HQ staff show a level of incompetence which is remarkable even by government standards", and also argued that an emerging social hierarchy where good jobs were going to those with chiefly status, rather than ability or training, was a deterrent to many (quoted in Naidu, 1997: 74). Such changes may also have reduced opportunities for further medical training.

Those who had chosen to remain in Fiji argued that 'job satisfaction' was the most significant influence, followed by 'lifestyle' (op cit: 69); although both categories are extremely vague, they do hint at some degree of altruism. On the other hand, but to a much lesser extent, there were stayers who believed their qualification would not be recognized abroad and others who felt they were too old to move, who remained for family reasons or who had a 'fear of the unknown'. Likewise, as one doctor indicated:

> Medical staff have to be compensated for their hard work especially after hours duty. At present work can be very stressful for those who are trying hard to improve the standards of health care. Why would one put in extra hours of work especially when they are underpaid? The 'good samaritan' and 'nightingale' days are over (quoted by Naidu, 1997: 78).

In other words, their rationale for staying was little to do with the situation in Fiji. Of those who had remained in Fiji, a third said they had no intention of migrating, over a quarter said they were keeping their options open, while a quarter had already lodged applications to migrate (op cit: 79-80). In contrast to much of the past 15 years in Fiji, this was a period of relative prosperity, a decade after the coups. Hence the high level of interest in emigration is exceptionally striking.

A second study undertaken in the same year analysed a balanced sample of 50 doctors throughout Fiji, in terms of their motivations should they decide to migrate in future (Azam, 1996). More than half (55%) emphasized the low salary as the primary source of dissatisfaction, followed by poor work conditions (41%) and the lack of postgraduate training (27%). Of rather lesser significance were a somewhat nebulous 'need' to migrate (18%), job dissatisfaction (14%), poor on-call allowance (9%) and the lack of malpractice insurance (5%). Broadly, therefore, the study emphasized economic issues as paramount, alongside specific problems attached to the job. However, these doctors remained in place and there is no indication of whether they were actually specifically contemplating migration or were willing to continue to cope with these problems. Hence the significance of their rationale for migration is uncertain.

One of the consequences of emigration is the replacement of local doctors with expatriates. In 1996, there was some concern that this was inappropriate, at least in the case of a group of Chinese doctors "whose training is allegedly doubtful, their oral English skills were very poor" and they may not have been examined for their skills before leaving China. Moreover "patients have also complained about difficulty in communicating with some expatriate doctors, especially Filipino, Burmese and Chinese doctors" (Naidu, 1997: 72). These claims of incompetence cannot be easily verified. Nonetheless, they are part of a perception that the health system is not providing an adequate service.

There was a greater probability that doctors in the private sector would not migrate, but "it seems that once a doctor resigns from the government he [sic] becomes an outcast' in that the public sector no longer sought to take any advantage of their skills" (Naidu, 1997: 77). There was then, greater scope for taking advantage of the private sector while working within the public sector.

Emigration remained a critical problem in 1999 when the Ministry of Health launched its own inquiry into the situation. At that time, there were vacancies for 78 doctors. It was then estimated that 78% of all the local doctors who had resigned in the previous 13 years had gone overseas (mainly to Australia, New Zealand and the United States of America). The remainder of those who had resigned were working in the private sector, mainly in the larger urban centres; hence rural areas have been particularly disadvantaged by these trends. Some 61% of those 302 doctors who had resigned were Fiji-Indians, while 12% were Fijians, 23% were expatriates and 4% were 'other'. Just over a third of all those who resigned left in the two post-coup years (1988 and 1989), with the largest subsequent numbers being in 1998 and 1999. Political instability was thus a critical catalyst to emigration.

Most of the doctors who had resigned in the 13-year period were in the 28-37 year age group, with the modal age being 31. In other words, these were the younger, and perhaps some of the better, doctors in the country. Some 65% of all doctors had resigned before completing five years service and the modal period was just three years. The majority of those who resigned were Principal Medical Officers, Senior Medical Officers and Medical Officers – the middle and lower grades – and it was strongly suggested that this was the result of a poor or limited career structure, unrealistic promotion criteria and the lack of recognition of doctors' hours of work and increased work pressures (Tuqa, 1999). It was emphasized that this migration had created problems for the health system.

The resignation and migration of doctors was seen to be a critical problem. First, it resulted in low quality health care and, second, it wasted much needed local resources through the 'brain drain' itself while requiring additional resources to maintain adequate health services. The shortage of human resources was already leading to inefficiency, low productivity, poor morale and greater frustration, a vicious circle that was only stimulating more migration. Equally, the absence of particular individuals was seen to be having a 'domino effect' through the under-utilization of other elements of the particular health facility (hospital wards, laboratories, etc).

The loss of SHPs was particularly a problem in rural areas where particular losses had clear effects, if they were not substitutable. Hence rural communities were increasingly choosing to bypass their official designated local clinics, to "fight all odds to attend [regional] hospital outpatient departments for medical consultations, even for their basic or minor health care problems" (Tuqa, 1999: 7). In a sense, rural problems became urban problems.

At every level, this is an uneconomic outcome: costly in time and money to the patients themselves and resulting in the under-utilization of rural health centres and congestion and inefficiency in the hospitals. At the rate of resignation that existed in 1999, when 23 doctors had resigned, the annual cost to the government was estimated to be around F$ 13 674 000 (US$ 7 000 000) in training costs at the FSM alone. Meanwhile, hiring of expatriate doctors cost an additional F$ 2 657 700 (US$ 1 400 000) per year, over and above what it would have cost to employ the same number of local graduates.

A series of attempts were made to discourage resignation and improve the health system, including, over a ten-year period, implementation of an improved salary structure, sponsored postgraduate training opportunities at the FSM, continuing education programmes, overseas attachments and twinning opportunities with overseas hospitals, locum practice for government doctors when they are on leave (so that they can earn some extra money). Such attempts at change also included private practice for specialists and consultants using government facilities after hours (so that they can earn some extra money), upgrading of subdivisional hospitals and health facilities (with more doctor positions being made available), improvement in the supply of drugs, stores and biomedical equipment to facilitate service delivery (and enable doctors to concentrate more on their key functions), decentralization of health management (giving peripheral staff more decision-making responsibility and accountability for their actions) and more transparency in staff promotions and transfers.

There has been no review of the specific success of implementing these policies, either collectively or individually. Nor is it clear how effectively they were implemented. However, the conclusion was drawn that "the above incentives, though comprehensive, seem to be largely ineffective as doctors continue to resign at the same rate through these years" (Tuqa, 1999: 9). Indeed, the rate of migration has increased over the past two years. That study therefore concluded that doctors should have been seen as a special case within the public service because of the long sustained nature of the shortage problem, its complexity and the socioeconomic costs of the shortage, and should have received substantially better remuneration within a new administrative structure that gave greater attention to promotion structures and training opportunities. Before the government could give these issues adequate consideration, the new political crises of 2000 intervened.

It is apparent that there have been problems for nurses too. The number of nurses who resigned increased rapidly in the three years before 1999, so that the output from the Fiji School of Nursing was only just keeping up with the number of those who had resigned or been redeployed (Tuqa, 1999). There has been considerable recent frustration among nurses over wages and conditions in the health service, irrespective of political and ethnic circumstances associated with events related to the 2000 coup. In mid-May 2000, the Fiji Nursing Association (FNA) organized a national strike, supported by about 1400 of 1600 nurses, which emerged from concern over allowances, overtime conditions and salaries in support of improved wages at all levels of the system. The government countered with a new pay scale somewhat less than that demanded by the FNA, but offered a review of minimum qualifications, fairer rostering, hardship allowances for nurses in remote areas, transport and uniform allowances. Though the Fiji Trade Union Congress did not support the strike, the principal national daily, *Fiji Times*, observed: "Everybody – even the Government – agrees that the nurses deserve better salaries and working conditions" and called on the government to meet the nurses demands (*Fiji Times*, 11 May 2000). While a starting salary, after four years training, of F$ 10 073 compared favourably with other nurse salaries in the region, it was perceived as comparing very unfavourably with the starting salaries of doctors in Fiji. The FNA criticized the Fiji Trades Union Congress on racial grounds (since the former was primarily Fijian and the latter Fiji-Indian) and the

Prime Minister for male chauvinism. The strike ended after three days when the national Permanent Arbitrator ruled in the nurses' favour.

Four days after the nurses' strike, a coup led by George Speight resulted in the Prime Minister and several members of the cabinet being held hostage for a month, and the country experiencing exceptionally difficult and tense times with the looting of stores, the collapse of several elements of the economy (notably tourism) and a significant rise in ethnic tensions. These tensions made social life extremely difficult, emphasized to Fiji-Indians that life was likely to remain difficult for them into the foreseeable future, and stimulated a rapid increase in the rate of emigration.

During 2000, a brief survey was undertaken of the changes of staffing in the small St Giles psychiatric hospital in Suva. During the 1997-2000 period, some 28 registered nurses and orderlies left the hospital: 24 of them left in the period before the coup. Of these, 19 left in search of better pay and improved conditions of work, three left because of changes in their personal relationships or marriage status, and two left for professional growth and development. Three were promoted or transferred elsewhere and one left for further education and training – these were not necessarily lost to the system. Eighteen of those who left went to New Zealand (where their nursing qualifications would be recognized), three went to Australia and one went to Palau. Over a short period of time, there was very substantial, and perhaps accelerating, attrition from one small hospital, with the bulk of those who left departing from the system and going overseas.

4.1.2 Doctors

The survey interviewed 20 local doctors and 64 local nurses based in Suva. Of the 20 doctors, the majority were in their 30s and early 40s, except for one 76-year-old who has been recalled from retirement. The lack of doctors in their 50s and 60s may be indicative of a trend for qualified doctors to migrate to work in other countries after becoming dissatisfied with the situation in their home country. Only seven of the 20 doctors were female and three quarters of the doctors were married (almost all had local spouses). Few doctors lived alone, while most had households containing spouses, children and often extended family such as parents, in-laws, grandchildren, aunts and uncles. It would seem likely that the role of the large extended family, and obligations to it, is a contributing factor for doctors who decide to remain in Fiji.

The reasons for entering the medical profession varied, with seven stating altruism as their main priority, five stating that income was a factor and only one person choosing to become a doctor to enable future migration. The availability of scholarships seems to have been a deciding factor for some, with four choosing the medical profession because of the educational opportunities offered to them. A further four chose medicine because of family tradition and three because of the prestige attached to the profession. As one doctor stated, "Top students go into medicine. Everybody looks up to you."

Although all of the doctors had studied in Fiji, half had left at some time previously for further study abroad (the most common destination being Australia). None had intended to move permanently at that time and only two had left the country for reasons other than their own study (one had parents who were missionaries in Burma for several years and one doctor's father was posted to Canada). One anaesthetist had worked in Adelaide and American Samoa, but only on clinical attachment supported by government, and had later returned to Fiji.

With regards to future migration, only four doctors were definitely planning to leave Fiji. Two of them have been offered jobs in Australia and the United States of America, lured by higher salaries and better research facilities. Three were leaving because of the political situation and each of them stated that they would prefer to stay but felt that there was no security for Fiji-Indian or non-Fijian families in Fiji following the coup. Six doctors were considering leaving temporarily to further their studies and gain exposure to new techniques and skills, but they all intended this to be a short-term prospect only and all wanted to return to Fiji. None of the doctors interviewed had returned from working overseas. This would seem to indicate that those doctors who leave Fiji to work abroad do not often return.

Twelve of the doctors interviewed had no desire to leave Fiji; 11 of them wanted to stay because "it's home". Having families and close friends in the country was another main reason for doctors wanting to remain. Several people felt a duty to stay and help their people and their country, sometimes because of financial assistance received. One doctor explained, "I was a sponsored student. I have a duty to serve the people of Fiji." Sometimes this sense of duty was simply from national pride: "The only reason for choosing to be a doctor is to work in Fiji and help my people in Fiji." One 37-year-old female doctor explained, "I've worked in Melbourne, but it seems that you are only doing it for the money. Here, you don't get much money, but you feel that you're really helping people." Doctors also seemed less likely to want to migrate if they owned land in Fiji, had no relatives abroad or were approaching retirement age.

All the doctors interviewed were employed on a full-time basis, with several on-call seven days a week. Salaries ranged from F$ 200 to F$ 996 a fortnight and averaged F$ 622. Although most doctors had received some type of regular pay increase in the past, approximately half specified having suffered a 12.5% pay cut following the 2000 coup, and the only benefit entitlement that they received was sick pay. Although the Fijian doctors interviewed voiced several concerns regarding the health service in Fiji, most enjoyed their profession, with 12 stating that they enjoy helping people and seeing patients recover, and five describing their work as challenging and interesting.

The main cause for complaint among the doctors interviewed related to pay structure and allocation of funds. Sixteen of the 20 specified insufficient shift allowances and set overtime allowance (rather than pro rata rates) in addition to the fact that doctors were graded the same way as other public servants. This was felt by them to be unacceptable due to the amount of training, hours worked and dedication required by doctors as opposed to other public servants. Administration and management issues were also high on the list of complaints, with nine doctors concerned about slow and inefficient delivery of requisitions ("Too much bureaucracy to approve simple, urgent requests. It's a major source of frustration for doctors"). Six felt that they had no support from management, and that the administrative structure was not supporting their endeavours.

Almost half of the doctors interviewed had serious concerns regarding promotion and the allocation of vacant positions. Although many doctors have annual reviews and appraisals, the general feeling was that these were not put to any practical use and that once a doctor has been put in place then there was no hope of progressing any further until a specific vacancy occurred (either through death or resignation). One doctor explained:

> Posts are for life until you are selected into a vacant high position. Promotions are supposedly on the basis of experience / seniority but not when decisions are made. ... There's a general sense of frustration – promotions are seen to be made on 'who you are' and 'who you know'. It's very disheartening for junior staff that people are promoted perhaps on the basis of years of service as opposed to quality of service.

Such complaints constantly recurred.

Seven of the doctors complained that no ongoing or further training was available and it was felt that there was no hope for progression within the present system without acquiring new skills. Clearly, the provision of ongoing or specialist training is difficult within the PICs where resources are limited and it can be difficult (or impossible) to find cover for a doctor while he or she is training overseas. One possible solution is to develop open learning courses as a way to provide more medical staff with the updated knowledge that they require. Not only would this alleviate the need for doctors to travel overseas for study, it is less likely that Fiji would lose medical personnel due to a combination of favourable overseas experiences and boredom and lack of job satisfaction at home.

Perhaps the most serious of all the concerns raised by the doctors was the perceived inequality of treatment between local and expatriate doctors.

Concerns ranged from differences in pay and allowances, the suitability of expatriates' previous experience and the appropriateness of the hiring procedures in place. As one doctor commented: "Recruitment of expatriates is often done without proper knowledge of the needs. For example, there are vacant positions that local doctors apply for, yet outsiders are being recruited for those positions – often without proper explanation to local doctors why they aren't given those vacant positions." The fact that expatriate doctors receive both gratuities and housing benefits was seen by many to be unfair to local doctors as was the fact that local doctors suffered a 12.5% pay cut following the 2000 coup, while expatriate doctors were unaffected. One doctor explained: "Expatriates are treated with favour compared to local doctors yet their performances are not up to standard. If only the same treatment for expatriates is given to local doctors, local doctors will be happy to hang in there for as long as the country needs them." When considering long-term solutions to staffing problems in Fiji, it is more appropriate to promote local staff to fill the vacant positions that they apply for and use the expatriate doctors to fill the gaps. In this way, the use of expatriate doctors would not create ill feeling between them and the local doctors, which results in yet more local personnel leaving the country.

Although 12 of the doctors interviewed for this study had no intentions of leaving Fiji, it is important to remember that they are the ones who have stayed and that many more doctors have already migrated. The doctors in this sample tended to have settled families in Fiji and generally had very few relatives abroad and so were less likely to leave, although even among those who were relatively settled, there were serious concerns expressed over the current situation in the Ministry of Health and more generally in the health system.

4.1.3 Nurses

Of the 64 Fijian nurses interviewed, the vast majority were female with ages fairly normally distributed from 23 to 60 years old. Some 49 nurses were married, often being part of extended families, and only two lived alone. All had attended nursing school in Fiji (although some received further training abroad.

Half of the nurses stated altruistic reasons for deciding to become nurses, while 12 entered the profession in order to care for their families. One nurse specifically entered nursing to "help the people in my village who were isolated from hospital" although, ironically, she was now living and working in an urban area of Fiji. Seven entered nursing through general interest or because they had enjoyed science in high school and five followed another family member into the medical profession. Four trained for a source of income and four because they "admired the uniforms". Most of the nurses had only ever trained and worked as nurses; only two had changed career (one was formerly a waitress and the other one, a cashier).

Eight of the nurses had lived abroad at some time previously; five left to pursue studies in New Zealand and Australia (three for themselves and two were accompanying studying spouses); two have been offered contracts abroad (Palau and Australia) and returned when the contract ended; and one nurse accompanied her husband when he was posted to Vanuatu for missionary work. All had positive feelings regarding their return. Those who had left on scholarships were bonded to return but were still happy to be reunited with family and friends, and those who had worked abroad were content to return once they had made the money they required.

Twenty-six nurses thought about working abroad at some stage in the future, all of them listing the chance to earn higher wages and get a better job as the main reasons for considering migration. The chance to work in a better institutional setting, and so have better opportunities for promotion and training, was also regarded as important. Several nurses considered moving overseas to further their education and that of their children. Of these 26, as many as 19 said they were actually intending to leave Fiji, although 10 were only intending to leave temporarily to earn extra money and planned to return. Almost all of those planning to leave were going to New Zealand and Australia (mostly due to the ease of transferring qualifications, family members already being settled there and familiarity due to previous visits). However, one nurse had a job offer in the United Kingdom and another in Saudi Arabia. One planned to go to the United States of America because of superior job opportunities and one wanted to retire there because Americans are "more friendly and outgoing". Three were leaving because of the recent coup and felt their future to be uncertain. Another was leaving because "nursing here is very generalized. I want to specialize." One nurse explained that she was leaving Fiji simply because there was "no incentive to stay".

By contrast, another 26 of the nurses had no plans to leave Fiji. Mostly their reasons for staying had to do with family, friends and being established in Fiji. Reasons such as having children in school, owning a good house and spouses having good jobs deterred most people from wanting to leave. Some people felt strong ties with their homeland and an obligation to stay. As one nurse declared, "Fiji needs us." One nurse would have liked to move abroad for the experience and chance to earn a better income, but her husband wanted to stay in Fiji and she refused to go alone. As she explained: "I have to be with my family. Money is not everything." Those reaching retirement age also had reservations about leaving, "Overseas life is very fast. We are too old to cope."

All the nurses questioned worked full-time with fortnightly salaries ranging from F$ 130 to F$ 456, with an approximate average of F$ 264. The majority received regular salary increases, although many of them have been affected by the 12.5% salary cut since the 2000 coup. Most received sick pay or paid annual leave, but only one nurse mentioned receiving any further training. When listing the positive aspects of their work, the nurses almost unanimously stated that it was the human aspect of their work that was important, such as helping others, meeting new people and working with colleagues.

Overwhelmingly, the main issues of dissatisfaction for nurses all centred around pay and work conditions and lack of career opportunities, with 35 complaining about the low salary and a further five about the lack of a shift allowance. Twenty-nine felt that they were overworked, particularly for the money they were paid, and nine felt that there was no incentive to do well. Some 33 nurses were dissatisfied with the lack of training they received and the situation where there was no adequate system in place to determine who could and should be eligible for training courses. As one nurse explained, "Nurses (are) sent on training when near retirement. Younger nurses should go as they have more years to serve." This feeling that only those approaching retirement benefited from training was echoed by many of the nurses. Another commented:

> [There is a] lack of support / encouragement from the Ministry for nurses who want to pursue further studies. Nurses, who go on further studies on leave without pay, or complete degree or diploma training, are taken back on the same salary scale they left on. There is no promotion / increment for studies completed, especially at their own expense. Nurses feel used and it frustrates them. Those who trained overseas tend to leave at some point.

Promotion was another important issue, with 15 nurses specifically stating that they felt promotions were dealt unfairly and based on favouritism as opposed to ability. One 60-year-old staff nurse commented on the "lack of transparency regarding promotion":

> Nurses are assessed every six months, yet nurses often do not get a promotion or increment for more than 10 years. Unless you are in the 'Good Book' or know someone upstairs, you are destined to remain a staff nurse for your entire career – no matter how hard you've worked and how well you have performed.

Issues of poor management and administration, including unfairness and nurses being posted to different departments regardless of training, were quoted by 11 of the nurses.

> Nurses with specialized training are often taken away to work in other units where they weren't trained. Nurses choose specialized areas and develop interest in specialized areas and train in specialized areas only to find that they are allocated to other units of no relevance to their training, interest and skills.

Issues like these are critical when examining skills migration, as people are rarely motivated by money alone. The fact that a large proportion of the nurses who were considering migration were drawn by the opportunity for better chances of promotion and training abroad indicates that this is very much the case within the nursing body of Fiji. Addressing issues of promotion, training and specialization are vital in retaining this workforce.

4.1.4 Expatriates

A small survey was carried out on expatriate doctors working in Fiji. Of the eight that took part, three were from Burma, with the remaining five hailing from such diverse locations as Hungary, Pakistan, the Philippines and Nigeria. All were working in government health clinics (two having worked in both rural and urban areas), and five have been in Fiji for over five years (two of those for more than 10 years). Half had previous overseas experience (apart from their country of origin), having worked in Australia, Estonia, Saudi Arabia, Libya and New Zealand.

Of the eight doctors who had come to work in Fiji, one had come to escape a coup in the home country, three had been posted by the United Nations and four had applied for jobs simply as a change, a chance to earn better wages or to reunite with family. None had been to Fiji previously and most seemed to have little knowledge about the country before arriving (most information having come from job offer letters, government agencies and travel books and brochures)

Income for the overseas doctors ranged from F$ 700 to F$ 1270 per fortnight and averaged approximately F$ 830 (this is some F$ 200 a fortnight above the average of local doctors' pay.) All received regular pay increases and housing benefits and five received a 25% annual income gratuity. One received subsidized transport and another received a utilities subsidy.

Most seemed fairly happy with their jobs in Fiji (three claiming they had no problems at all). Dissatisfaction with the working environment included the uncertainty of working on a contract, lack of equipment and specialist training, low pay, being moved around between departments and one mentioned some racial abuse from patients. The only problems reported regarding living in the country itself were the political situation, particularly the recent coup, and the inability to put down roots because of contract work.

Seven of the doctors were working on contracts and five of those planned to extend their contract periods. Their reasons for staying included stability and the wish to continue their children's education without disruption. Of those leaving, one doctor's husband had not found work in Fiji and wanted to return to employment and another wished to return home to begin a private practice. Five of the eight doctors intended to leave Fiji eventually and none of those had plans to return in future years.

Unfortunately, due to the small sample size of this group, it is impossible to draw any conclusive information regarding expatriate doctors in Fiji, although it would appear that several remain for a fairly long-term period and seem relatively happy with conditions there. There is no clear indication of the extent to which they contribute to the health care system.

4.1.5 The power of politics

The widespread rise in emigration in the last two years was strongly evident in the health sector, not only in the Ministry's statistics, but also in the attitudes of those remaining in the system. This was so to the extent that it was remarked upon in several newspaper articles as being perhaps the sector most affected by emigration. Two months after the 2000 coup, a newspaper article entitled, "Flight of doctors deals a body blow to the system" (Appendix 2), drew attention to the flight of Fiji-Indian doctors, part of a larger brain drain that also included nurses, teachers and accountants, with five doctors having notified their intention to resign in the previous week, and the 'nation's health system approaching an abyss' to the extent that Ministry officials were about to leave for the Philippines with the intention of recruiting 48 doctors there. Fiji had turned to the Philippines rather than other sources since one impact of the coup was a 12.5% pay cut imposed across the whole of the public service.

It was also claimed that a further impact of the coup, and the resultant emigration, was a decline in health services especially in rural areas. There was evidence of inadequate diagnoses and the lack of timely treatment, and the impending winding up of the postgraduate medical school, because of the impossibility of retaining skilled high level teaching staff, and where there had already been three resignations (Brown, 2000a). A subsequent article drew attention to the migration of a Fiji-Indian doctor who had eventually moved to Australia, where many of his relatives had already moved, because of the fear and insecurity that followed the coup: "It is not good enough to have all the money in the world and at the end of the day be worried you are going to be robbed and bashed. I am leaving with reluctance. I have known the Fiji way of life. I would love to stay in Fiji, because when you [are] 40 you are well settled" (quoted in Brown, 2000b). Political crises thus affected even older, established doctors. While the coup was a single political event, its racial overtones and the economic crisis that it engendered had a particularly destructive effect on the health system, especially among doctors, where the proportion of Fiji-Indians was higher than elsewhere in the health service.

Among nurses, a high proportion of whom were Fijian, the situation that followed the coup was less devastating. Nonetheless, migration was one outcome. As early as June 2000, the Fiji Nurses Association (FNA) was seeking to hold meetings with the Ministry to develop plans to counter the shortage of nurses, at a time when Cabinet had just supported proposals to expand the responsibilities of nurse practitioners into clinical areas of nursing practice, allow part-time employment for nurses who have been out of the service for various reasons, increase the number of ward assistants to relieve nurses of non-core nursing duties and allow them to focus on nursing, and develop a new development campus for the Fiji School of Nursing at Lautoka (the second largest city in Fiji).

Even so, by September 2000, less than four months after the coup, some 50 nurses had resigned, with several being offered jobs either in the private sector or in New Zealand. During the same period, 45 nurses had emigrated, 32 of those being Fiji-Indians and 13 Fijians. They had been offered jobs in New Zealand, the Marshall Islands, Cook Islands and Palau. Another large group were in Saipan (Northern Marianas). The Fiji Nurses Association was concerned about the loss and claimed that the remaining nurses were "overworked and underpaid [and] are refusing to work overtime because they are stressed out. They love their profession and they go out of their way to give their best to their patients." The FNA recommended that the government restore the 12.5% reduction in salaries because "to increase the intake, or to extend the retirement age will not solve the problem" (*Fiji Times*, 9 September 2000, 11 September 2000). The events preceding the coup, that is the strikes in favour of superior wages and benefits, are evidence that there were already discontents in the sector prior to the coup. However, the dramatic political events proved to be a catalyst to an equally dramatic and continuing process of emigration that has very substantially weakened one of the more effective health care systems in the region. While the coup can scarcely be regarded as trivial, it effectively drew attention to the manner in which political and social unrest could easily contribute to the selective migration of the highly skilled.

4.1.6 Migrants and destinations

Emigration from Fiji occurred before that in most other Pacific island countries, being well underway in the 1960s. Much of that early migration included relatively skilled migrants, most of who were Fiji-Indians moving to Canada, Australia and New

Zealand. As early as 1971, the costs of a skill drain had already been recognized in terms of training needs:

> There are long gestation periods involved in many types of professional, technical and vocational skill training and in the short run the output of these skills cannot be radically changed. In the next few years, despite special and temporary government measures to circumvent or mitigate the problems the combination of the emigration of skilled and trained manpower, inadequate training facilities and insufficient numbers of skilled people estimated to be in the pipeline...will together contribute to a deterioration of the skilled manpower situation with most serious shortages occurring in the supply of technicians and qualified tradesmen (Ward 1971: 236).

This selective movement was becoming so substantial that it was possible to conclude almost two decades ago that "the most striking conclusion on the impact of international migration from Fiji is that it constitutes a very substantial skill and brain drain" (Connell, 1985: 24). In 1974, a special study was undertaken of the skill drain from Fiji, which made recommendations for the provision of more appropriate and cheaper training courses in Fiji, that would not meet international criteria, the introduction of bonding for students, the payment of an 'emigration tax' and the repayment of the public costs of post-primary education (Bartsch, 1974: 7). Other than bonding, these suggestions were generally not put into practice. Such trends were then only incipient elsewhere, and no other Pacific government had yet expressed concern about skill losses.

Skilled migration was highly selective. In the years after independence Fiji-Indians already felt themselves to be 'strangers in their own land' and migration was selectively of Fiji-Indians. Between the 1960s and the end of the 1980s, Fiji lost around 100 000 citizen overseas and almost 30% of them went during the two post-coup years, 1988 and 1989. More importantly, within a year of the coups, about a third of the health workforce had emigrated, involving ancillary, nursing and medical staff, and including 160 doctors, almost all of whom were Fiji-Indians (Lander and Miles, 1992: 29). Until that point, almost all emigrants had been Fiji-Indians; however, in the wake of the coups, a new movement of Fijians became evident. As elsewhere, but particularly for Tonga and Samoa, this has meant that there are large numbers of migrants overseas and that these migrants can be a key influence on subsequent migration patterns.

The migration of skilled health workers has long been part of the process of emigration, but has accelerated in recent years, partly because of increased recruitment within Fiji. Despite an informal agreement between countries in the region not to encourage the immigration of health personnel from nearby island states, this has been a practice for some time. The Marshall Islands and Nauru (with only one indigenous skilled health worker) have long recruited Fijian nurses, who often went on contracts of several years for the experience and substantially greater incomes; in the Marshall Islands, the average nursing salary is three times that in Fiji (personal communication, 2000). Palau has more recently begun to recruit Fijian nurses, as has New Zealand. In 1999, a newspaper article entitled, "Nurses chase New Zealand jobs" (*Fiji Times*, 3 June 1999), stated that more than 70 nurses had attended specially established interviews designed to attract nurses to New Zealand. The United Kingdom was also recruiting Fijian clinical nurses at the same time. Thus a greater and more visible active recruitment of Fiji nurses has occurred at a time when it has become more difficult to retain nurses because of dissatisfactions with wages, conditions of employment and political circumstances.

4.1.7 New Zealand

The 1996 survey of doctors who had migrated to New Zealand recorded a combination of economic, political and educational influences on migration. New Zealand was generally perceived as a politically stable country where there were opportunities for socioeconomic advancement in terms of better salaries, working conditions, better education for children and a higher standard of living. It was pointed out that doctors who had emigrated had well demonstrated their ability to succeed at higher levels in the system, though such promotion opportunities may have been denied to them in Fiji. These key factors were also influenced by the possibility of family reunions, previous overseas experience, the wishes of spouses and children and prior citizenship of the destination. This migration also represented something of a skill loss; one respondent, a shopkeeper, had used his status as a doctor "to acquire a New Zealand medical license but chose to become a shopkeeper instead. He said that his career mattered less to him than the fact that a variety of tertiary educational opportunities were now accessible to his children" (Naidu, 1997: 69). While this latter example is somewhat exceptional, it does indicate that there are very powerful influences on migration that have little directly to do with health issues.

4.1.8 Australia

Since the mid-1980s, Australia has been the principal destination of Fiji-Indians migrating from Fiji. By 1996, there were over 20 000 Indo-Fijians over the age of 15 in the country, many of whom had formal qualifications. These included a number of nurses and doctors. A sample of nine nurses and doctors were interviewed in Sydney as part of the present study. All were Fiji-Indians. Their average age was 50 and the majority had been in Australia for more than a decade. They had entered the health profession for a variety of reasons, though altruism, the prospects of a good income and family enthusiasm were key reasons. One who came from a high status public service background became a doctor because only law and medicine were perceived as being appropriate. Rather differently, the sole nurse was encouraged by her family so that she could look after them in their old age. Only one, a blood collector who had migrated in 2000, was not employed at a relatively high level since she had failed the Australian medical exam.

Unlike the 1996 migrants in New Zealand, most of the Fiji-Indians in Sydney stated reasons other than politics to explain their migration, but political considerations were usually present in part. For two thirds of the migrants, education was the principal reason for migration, partly for their children and partly for themselves. At least two had been sent to Australia for further education; one had met her husband there and never returned; the 1987 coups intervened while the other was in Australia and he too chose not to return. Several moved for family reasons, such as to accompany a wife or husband or, in one case, because more of her kin were in Australia than Fiji. Coups were specifically mentioned by three people, one of whom had had his business firebombed in 1987 and had migrated to Australia via New Zealand. At least two would never have left Fiji without the political unrest. In almost every case, migration had been a collective decision, most obviously when parents were sending their children to Australia for education. Not a single person stated that they had migrated for superior employment opportunities or because the work they had been doing in Fiji was unsatisfying or inadequately paid.

In terms of why the respondents have gone to Australia rather than elsewhere, few appeared to have considered another destination, but more than half have gone because of having kin in Australia, and three had essentially established their own connections through their education there. Only one specifically suggested that it was the salary in Australia that was the primary motive. (Implicit in this, but specifically stated by only one respondent, was that Australia's migration requirements were relatively easy to meet.) Out of this rather small sample, the primary causes of migration were thus less to do with employment (though that may have been implicit in several cases) but primarily linked to their children's future or that of the entire household, and were much influenced by the location of kin. However, because of the political uncertainties of Fiji, and the long duration of this particular group in Australia, they may have been relatively exceptional.

Not one of the interviewees had any intention of returning to Fiji. Few mentioned that political changes might at least make them think about returning. Several had become Australian citizens, had sold their property in Fiji or had no remaining relatives there; one who still visited regularly stated that he had become an Australian citizen to ensure his protection when he returned. In the sense that few expected ever to return, despite intermittent nostalgia, Fiji-Indians are unlike other Pacific island migrant groups who rarely rule out the possibility of return.

This group of Fiji-Indians were perhaps unusual in their relative longevity of residence in Australia (and in Sydney). More recent migrants, and specifically several of the doctors who moved to Australia after the 2000 coup, have tended to live in Queensland, where it is relatively easy to find medical appointments quickly.

4.1.9 Canada

A small sample of five Fiji-Indians was interviewed in Vancouver, Canada. Although one nurse had migrated in 1997, none of the others had migrated after 1975; hence they were an unusually well established group, even more so than those in Sydney. The youngest was 43. None cited political issues (other than perhaps 'land disputes') as a reason for migration. Most had moved to Canada for a range of reasons, including inadequate educational opportunities for themselves and their children, lack of satisfying work opportunities (including not working at full potential) and the possibility of advanced education in Canada.

None intended to return to Fiji. One was uncertain, but would only contemplate migration "if political stability made it possible to retire there". Another noted that Fiji needed "education based on merit and ability, not on race or who you know" to enable a real prospect of significant return migration. Others were too well established in Vancouver, with families who had grown up there, and often with other kin there rather than in Fiji; one doctor also had a real estate business, and several had paid off their homes. As elsewhere, the prospects for significant Fiji-Indian return migration to Fiji were poor.

4.2 PALAU

Palau is the smallest of the PICs included in this study, with an economy that is largely dependent on American aid, and some degree of tourism. It has a population of about 19 000, who mostly live in the urban centre of Koror. About a third of the population are on distant outlying islands with a very small number on very distant coral atolls to the south of the main archipelago.

The health care system of Palau is largely centralized around an 80-bed hospital in Koror that was opened in 1992. The Ministry of Health staff in 1998 included 22 medical officers, three dental officers and 87 registered and licensed nurses. Although expatriates then represented less than 7% of all employees in the health service, they included seven medical officers, two of the three dental officers, the one pharmacist in the Ministry of Health and six nurses. At that time, "wages and benefits in Palau [were] not competitive with those of the Northern Marianas [Saipan], resulting in many Palauan nurses staffing Northern Marianas facilities, while Palau recruits from Fiji and Asia to maintain essential services" (UNDP, 1998: 118). In more recent years, Palau has continued to recruit nurses, and a growing number and proportion of the nurses are from overseas, especially from Fiji.

Palau has also implemented plans to reduce nursing shortages by establishing a Nursing School at the Palau Community College. The school enrolled its first intake of 13 students in 1998, at a time when the economy had 'a critical shortage' of interregional nurses. Students can graduate at four levels, from Palauan Practical Nurse through to United States Registered Nurse. The extent to which students will choose the longer and more demanding latter course – and perhaps move on to the United States of America – remains to be seen. The attrition rate of nurses would be reduced by the establishment of a nursing incentive and clinical career ladder, based on performance evaluations and identified competencies. Similarly, the ability of nurses to progress in nursing could be facilitated by recognition of advanced or specialized nursing competencies.

Palau has found it more difficult to produce medical practitioners, a situation that is more generally true of Micronesia. Secondary educational institutions produce few students who could qualify for the courses of either Pacific or metropolitan Pacific Rim medical schools. Few of those who have gone to the Fiji School of Medicine have graduated. About 15 Micronesians (from Palau, the Federated States of Micronesia and the Marshall Islands) graduated from the University of Hawaii School of Medicine between 1970 and 1990, but the majority remained in the United States of America. The majority of doctors in the region continue to be expatriates, despite the establishment of the Pacific Basin Medical Officer Training Program on Pohnpei (the Federated States of Micronesia) in the late 1980s (Dever, 1991). Palau's goal is to provide specialist training for selected Palauan doctors in order to reduce national dependency on expatriate specialists.

4.2.1 Nurses and doctors

The survey data indicate that expatriates hold a high proportion of posts within the health service. This is because there have been inadequate numbers of Palauan graduates rather than because of emigration or other forms of attrition. However, most of the Palauans working there intended to remain; many simply responded that this was their home country, and this was where they had their home, kin and friends. One surgeon valued the opportunity to combine medicine with farming and fishing. Some couched this in altruistic terms, including "to do good", "to help my country people" or "to participate in nation-building" (as one stated after being away for 28 years). Most of these were relatively old.

From a small sample of seven doctors, women seemed most likely to consider migration either because of "too much politics in the Ministry of Health", "benefits and promotion for the few" or to find a more supportive environment for psychiatric medicine. Others too were also conscious of local problems – "uncaring management", "the usual problems of management/supervision, politics, etc.", "unequal opportunities and salaries" and more general problems of morale and overwork. Men appeared more likely to cope with these disadvantages perhaps because they were more easily able to surmount them. For a small nation, Palau has an exceptional degree of factionalism and bitterness in the political sphere (that has posed serious problems in the past).

It is improbable that the health care system is not also politicized, to the detriment of effective management.

Palauan nurses were even more likely to express a wish to remain in the Palauan health system, especially where they were close to retirement. Many too were altruistic: "I generally like this job – helping people, especially sick people;" and "It's my country and I work to help my people." A 29-year-old female nurse who has spent four years being educated at the FSM summarized it well: "Well, first of all it is my home country and I feel I owe it to the Palauans that I stay and work for them, even though sometimes it gets frustrating. But I can cope with it, and of course my family and relatives are here." One had returned after 25 years away "to be close to relatives and my beloved homeland". Once again it is the presence of kin that ties people to their home country. Not a single one of the 10 Palauan nurses sought to go overseas, though almost all had some degree of frustration with the system, citing: "not enough nurses to take care of sick patients", "low salary and nurses don't show up on time", "no promotion" and "high levels of stress". Because of some of these reasons, Palau has sought overseas nurses to fill the shortage.

Overall, both Palauan nurses and doctors generally intended to remain and seemed likely to do so despite their intermittent or long-term frustrations. Some of those problems, such as the lack of support for specialist services such as psychiatry, are never likely to be easily supported in very small states such as Palau (which also has the advantage of being able to refer cases to Guam). However, other Palauan doctors and especially nurses have already left.

4.2.2 Expatriates

The expatriate doctors in Palau were exceptionally diverse. Of the nine participants in the survey, two were from the United States of America and there was one each from Burma, the Philippines, Fiji, Solomon Islands, the Republic of Korea, the Federated States of Micronesia (Chuuk) and Vanuatu. While a few had married Palauans, the remainder had come under contracts of varying duration. Some had no idea where Palau was; others had some general knowledge. Many of them appeared to cope with the system no worse than their Palauan counterparts, but that might be due to some degree of altruism or reluctance to criticize an alien system.

Only those expatriates who came from elsewhere in the Pacific (including the Philippines) stated that they had come for financial reasons; others found the salary levels somewhat inadequate. Several experienced frustration with the system: "lack of equipment", "very difficult to supervise and manage programmes", "high medical costs", "overwork" and "medical-legal litigation problems". However, one who enjoyed the wages and working conditions claimed that he had been so successful that he "helped improve the health care system to a satisfactory level comparable with Hawaii". Others were more sanguine about their efforts and several referred to loosely cultural problems: "don't speak the language", "sense of entitlement makes me feel unappreciated", "the problems of being a non-citizen", and "the many languages spoken, hard to understand their English". Not surprisingly, the doctors nonetheless generally felt that they were coping, though few intended to stay for many years in Palau. Since none of the Palauans commented on their expatriate counterparts, there is no indication if the cultural differences were significant in the actual delivery of health services.

The situation was somewhat similar for the migrant nurses. Of the 13 in the sample, one had come from the neighbouring Federated States of Micronesia to join his wife, one had come from Vanuatu, another was on a contract from the Japan International Cooperation Agency (JICA), and the remainder had been contracted from Fiji. Ironically, the migrant from the Federated States of Micronesia originated from one of the remote Outer Islands of the State, and had become a nurse "since the profession was badly needed on the island". The Fijian nurses, all of whom were females of Fijian ethnicity, had come in some part for the much superior wages, but they usually also expressed other reasons, most of which could be summarized as the desire to taste new experiences: "I actually became a nurse so that I could travel", "the travel experience", "better education opportunities". Many had become nurses as much for the financial and other rewards as out of any degree of altruism. Sometimes their families had encouraged them in this direction, for the monetary rewards, although just as many had been warned away by their families because of the poor incomes and the stress. They were therefore a mixed group, but few were younger than their mid-30s.

The Fijian nurses were a particularly well-trained group. All were Intensive Care Unit nurses; hence the loss to Fiji was substantial. They were recruited from the Lautoka and Suva areas in Fiji, by word of mouth and personal connections, rather than by advertisement, and were interviewed in Fiji. They were selected because of their skills, in preference to Filipina nurses, who commanded lower wages but experienced some discrimination in Palau (Dever G, personal communication, 1999). They were normally recruited on three- to five-year contracts.

Most of the nurses had gained some benefits from the experience of working in Palau although several discovered that the high wages were offset by high costs of living, in a country where much food is imported. However, the few who had considered the possibility of staying beyond their contract period only intended to remain for the income. Some had gained new experiences and skills "working with visiting United States medical teams" and "learning to be flexible and adapt new techniques", and several enjoyed working with their new patients and in different conditions. For some, the new experiences were less pleasant. One listed a series of problems, such as "too many non-nursing duties" and "the high cost of living and the lack of social activities".

Once again cultural issues were evident, notably in language issues; several of the expatriate nurses referred to a language barrier and raised the issue of whether "English should be spoken in the workplace". It is impossible to indicate whether the frequently referred to cultural differences were reflected in the actual delivery of health care. Since the nurses were selected from a wider group of applicants, these cultural differences might have been expected to be rather less significant.

The intended return to their home countries of most of the expatriate doctors and nurses, after their contracts had been completed, is indicative of some of the difficulties that Palau has in obtaining an adequate health workforce on the basis of migration, while the extent of cultural differences certainly indicates that this might not necessarily be the best way of dealing with sometimes subtle health requirements. At the same time, grandiose claims apart, the fact that several nurses referred to the lack of professionalism of their local counterparts, and that they had been selected from a larger pool and thus were likely to be particularly competent, suggests that they might have had (or at least had the potential to have) some limited success in raising treatment standards. Without other data from Palau such conclusions cannot be adequately made. It is however clear that Palau will have to rely in part on a migrant health workforce for some years to come and that this might not be easy to achieve in the future.

4.3 SAMOA

Samoa (formerly Western Samoa) is one of the larger Polynesian island states, with a population of about 170 000, two thirds of which are on the island of Upolu, which contains the only town, Apia, and the National Hospital. Samoa has a small open economy, dependent on a narrow resource base – centred on agriculture and fishing – and also on aid and remittances from overseas migrants.

Samoa has a health system that has been substantially affected by the large-scale emigration of trained personnel. "While there have been significant numbers of Samoan doctors trained since independence, losses of doctors to other countries in the region and to [the Pacific] rim countries continues to be a major problem". Hence, in 1991, most Samoan doctors in the public system were largely of retirement age (15 out of 34) or new graduates (8 of the 34 being aged less than 35) and accounted for only 60% of all public sector doctors, with most of the remainder being United Nations Volunteer doctors. Several doctors had actually been brought back from retirement to cope with the shortage (World Bank, 1994: 315). This unusually skewed age distribution has not substantially changed since then.

It was argued at the start of the 1990s that "many new graduates have not been satisfied with salaries offered and have acquired more remunerative positions elsewhere. According to one 1992 estimate, some 50 per cent of medical graduates migrated over the period 1958-1991 with 80 per cent of this loss occurring since 1980" (cited in World Bank, 1994: 322). Similar problems of retention were evident for other skilled categories of staff such as pharmacists and dentists (and outside the health sector), and were simply assumed to be "due to salary levels offered by the government relative to alternative employment opportunities in the region and rim countries" (op cit: 323-4). By contrast, the number of nurses was then regarded as adequate, though there was a shortage by 1998 when there were only 140 nurses working at the National Hospital (compared with the required staff number of 168). Since then this situation has not improved.

At about the same time, it was noted that the provision of services in remote and rural areas was particularly inadequate and that those who were working in remote areas had limited contact with the centre and felt excluded from the health care system. "Staff development in distant areas is not happening and needs to be addressed. Most of the nurses work alone and have no access to medical personnel so they really need to upgrade their skills and knowledge. A decent salary should be a good motivation for people to do the training and then stay in the remote areas. Accommodation for the nurses should be upgraded to enhance her [sic] job satisfaction. This should include providing all necessities" (Kerslake, 1993: 92-96). In essence, the shortage of personnel was most acute in rural areas and those who worked there felt isolated and ignored; there was some considerable probability that this was affecting the standard of health care there.

In order to slow the migration of doctors, the World Bank recommended that the Samoan government would probably need to raise the pay and benefits through the "judicious granting of allowances over and above base salaries which link the rewards of doctors to work loads and health system needs" and argued that the exact nature of such a system would have to be determined empirically and "be related to future options for migration" so that the actual remuneration of professionals (including doctors) working long hours and on night shifts would not be limited by reference to salary points in the public service but be related to actual scarcities and needs (World Bank, 1994: 336). That complex and detailed formulation is indicative of the concern attached to migration, and of the complexities of actually resolving the question. There is no evidence that Samoa was able, or even sought, to put such a complex recommendation into practice.

Since the early 1990s, there has been a continued migration of doctors, and some parallel migration of nurses, but the migration of doctors appears to have slowed. That may have been as a result of a decision taken a decade ago to centre all training of medical officers at the Fiji School of Medicine. The perception was that training at FSM was more appropriate and cheaper, and "there was a lower propensity for graduates to emigrate to rim countries relative to graduates of rim country institutions" (World Bank, 1994: 322). Whether that has proved to be true remains to be seen. Certainly in 1998 the shortage of doctors remained a problem. The World Bank then further recorded:

> One of the chief problems of the health system is the shortage of trained health personnel – especially doctors, specialist nurses, pharmacists, laboratory technicians – positions that require extensive education. ... Poor management, weak supervision and lack of satisfactory training further compound this problem. Low public salaries make it difficult for Samoa to retain trained medical staff. Many staff move to the private sector or emigrate in search of higher remuneration. Attrition is particularly damaging when public funds are used to train personnel who later leave the public sector (World Bank, 1998: 18).

At that time, over 40% of the doctors who remained in the public sector were above retirement age, and there were no overseas doctors since the recruitment programme had been phased out because it was concluded that the programme was a deterrent to the government devising a permanent solution to the problem. Special tabulations produced from the 1999 Samoan statistical data revealed that just three nurses had moved overseas in the previous year (but that may be the tip of an iceberg since there was no onus on those who left to declare an occupation from which they had resigned or retired) and no doctors had moved.

In 2000, there were 43 medical officers in the public health service sector in Samoa and, though there were 10 vacancies, this represented a substantial improvement from the situation a decade earlier since the population of Samoa had scarcely changed (because of general ongoing emigration). The private sector had also grown over the same time period. Almost all the doctors were Samoans. By contrast, the number of nurses was almost unchanged from the start of the decade, having declined slightly from 251 to 248 over that time period, and there were several vacancies.

Just one doctor and a handful of nurses were officially posted at the second national hospital on the island of Savai'i (larger in size but with less than half the population of the main island). Savai'i was therefore without obstetrics specialization or a surgeon. The resident doctor was a young man whose family had remained in the capital. He was described by a senior public servant in the Department of Health as "serving about 200 people a day, an enormous burden for a young graduate. Since he is always on call he sees his family about once a month. While remote folk believe their work will be recognized, it is not. They are effectively out of sight and out of mind" (personal communication, 2000). Not only is this indicative of an unusually inequitable situation where the health needs of just under 30% of the population are being relatively poorly served – and thus reasonably typical of circumstances elsewhere in the region – but it is also indicative of a situation where such an individual may be unlikely to stay long (either there or within the country) unless it is quite clear that there are reasonable promotion prospects.

The shortage of doctors has meant that some procedures could not be undertaken in Samoa. As a result, overseas referrals were relatively commonplace, e.g. for cardiac problems. It was estimated that the cost of oversees referrals was as much as 20% of the health budget (personal comm., 2000). In addition, various procedures could not be undertaken on Savai'I; hence there were also costly transfers from that island (a not unfamiliar situation in the region). In March 2000, a team of American eye surgeons were working in Savai'i where they had undertaken 33 eye operations (again a rather familiar situation in the region).

A significant shift of doctors to the private sector occurred following the opening of a new MedCen private medical centre in Apia, and it was suggested that these included the better doctors from the public sector. Costs of consultation at MedCen were approximately 10 times those of the public sector (though, in a new hospital, facilities were somewhat superior). The hospital has sought accreditation to Australian standards (Polu, 1999: 12). Nurses too had moved from the public to the private sector, both to MedCen and to a private school for American students: "Nurses from the National Hospital have been attracted to the school because of the good salaries it offers. This became a concern for the health authorities who kicked up a lot of fuss over the issue" (Fatupaito, 1997: 21). About 12 nurses work at the school on salaries upward of T$ 540 a fortnight, very much more than the standard wage in the public sector. The loss of skilled personnel from the public sector is therefore somewhat predictable, where superior wages and superior conditions exist in the same place.

While there was no evidence that the migration of nurses had substantially increased during the decade (and the official records indicate few emigrants) there has been considerable recent unrest among the nursing profession over what were perceived as poor wages and conditions. A strike threat from the Samoa Nurses Association (SNA) early in 2000, with widespread support from the Public Services Association (PSA) and the Samoan Trades Union Congress, did not ultimately secure a 5% pay rise (that other unions sought for all government employees). The existing base salary was T$ 7395 (US$ 2000) for a nurse with a three-year nursing diploma. As an article in the *Samoa Observer* recorded at the time, their claim "was more than demanding a fair wage. It is about respect for one's position and a call for just and fair treatment for the public service in general. And they have a fair argument ... when your starting salary is between $7-8000 that immediately puts off people in future generations aspiring to this all important position" (Rees, 2000). Crucial to the nurses' concerns were wages, but the conditions of employment were also in question.

In response to the strike threat, the Minister of Health commented that nurses had more claim to a pay increase than others in the public service: "There is a fundamental flaw in the logic that a Diploma is a Diploma! The duties and hardships of nursing are unique to the nursing profession. If the nurses successfully negotiate a $9045 per annum starting salary for those with a Diploma in Nursing, all other Diploma holders think they are entitled to the same salary. They need to set up Task Forces, Committees and spend three years negotiating their own package just as the nurses did" (quoted in *Samoa Observer*, 7 May 2000). In justification of the demand for increased wages the SNA pointed out that there was a very significant nursing shortage (in that 300 were working but 400 were needed); hence family members had to attend to sick relatives in hospital, nurses consistently had to work overtime, the demands being such that many had moved overseas or gone to work in private businesses. The PSA stated that a survey conducted three years earlier by the Division of Nursing showed that most of those who had gone overseas were younger nurses, who had gone for training and better opportunities: "The bottom line is money. Just like doctors, according to an NUS [National University of Samoa] official' (ibid).

At the same time, the PNA secured a change in status for the Diploma in Nursing, which would become a three-year Bachelor's Degree in Nursing, to be introduced at the National University of Samoa in 2001. Concerns remained that the wage was still inadequate as a starting salary for those who had undergone three years of training and that it would not be enough to attract an adequate number of nurses into the profession. Equally, it is highly likely that graduates of the course could easily gain New Zealand registration and thus migrate. The long and unsuccessful struggle to improve a reasonably low salary, and the Minister's rather lukewarm response to the nurses' concerns (and those of others in the public sector) with wages and morale, is indicative of the challenges to improving conditions in this part of the public sector (despite the Minister's implicit recognition that the claims of nurses were superior to those of others). While upgrading training, at least in nomenclature, is likely to minimally improve the status of nurses, it may also make their qualifications more transferable.

The wage and salary problems are part of a situation where Samoa, like most other Pacific island countries, has no human resource plan for the health sector and, at the same time, wages and salaries constitute 60% of the costs of the Department of Health. Nor is there any career development structure for medical officers, which would both provide sufficient staff and ensure that they had the necessary experience and skills to undertake higher-level functions as posts become vacant. In the absence of such a career structure, doctors "believe that working in the National Hospital is the only option that will ensure promotion within the Department of Health" (World Bank, 1998: 19). This emphasizes the problems attached to adequately serving the needs of remote areas.

The World Bank therefore concluded that the Department needed a human resource plan that would "provide incentives that will improve staff performance, including attractive salaries, benefits such as in-service training programmes linked to salary increments, well-structured career development paths and performance based rewards and sanctions for improper referral. Health professionals must be given remuneration packages including a benefit package and bonuses should be based on labour market conditions" (World Bank, 1998: 19). Once again, as in Fiji, what was being recommended was extremely complex, and almost certainly incapable of being monitored even if acted upon, in the familiar small island state situation of limited numbers of middle-range management professionals.

4.3.1 Doctors

The current survey interviewed 34 nurses and 15 doctors in Samoa. Of the doctors, 10 were male and five were female, with four in their 20s, four in their 30s, three in their 40s, two in their 50s and one in their 60s. This could indicate that doctors are migrating once they reach their late 30s and early 40s. As elsewhere, this is of particular concern since these doctors are highly likely to be experienced and so represent a great loss to the system. An alternative reason could be that many newly qualified doctors left Samoa some time ago, which would account for the lack of numbers in the older age groups. Three quarters of the doctors were married (most with children), and four lived with their parents and other extended family members. Most had studied to medical school level, with four having completed postgraduate studies. Most doctors had completed at least some of their studies overseas, the most common destination being Fiji, followed by Papua New Guinea, New Zealand and one in American Samoa.

The reasons for entering the profession varied but most claimed to have studied medicine for altruistic motives. Influence from families was evident, with nine mentioning that their family had influenced their decision to some degree and one claimed that his family wanted him to be a doctor to "uplift family status and standing in the community". Prestige and status was felt to be important by four of the respondents and a further six entered the profession for the monetary rewards. The majority of the doctors were employed in urban hospitals, although some had had a variety of positions in rural and urban health clinics and urban private practices.

Of the 11 who had lived away from Samoa, nine had gone abroad for further education (their own, their spouse's or a parent's). Study destinations included New Zealand, Fiji, Australia and Papua New Guinea.

Two had left on temporary attachment for work experience (to Solomon Islands, American Samoa and Niue). The majority chose these destinations because of educational opportunities there (or had their destination dictated by the terms of their scholarship). Most were happy to have returned to Samoa, mainly through an attachment to their home country and the desire to remain with friends and relatives. Three were contractually bound to return because of a bonded scholarship but were happy to return in any case. Only one doctor regretted the decision to return, finding the working conditions in Samoa difficult: "First, the pay is lousy (overworked and underpaid). Second, this is my first year as junior registrar and I have been appointed to a post with a lot of responsibilities and been deprived of a lot of sleep."

Two thirds of the Samoan doctors had considered moving abroad at some point in the future (generally to earn some extra money and continue their studies), and half were actually intending to migrate (mostly in the next 2 to 3 years). Most of those moving abroad were intending to live in New Zealand because friends and family were already settled there. One doctor argued, "I have many relatives there. It's like staying home." The existence of a large Samoan population in New Zealand was also a factor, with one doctor describing a need for Pacific island doctors to service the needs of the community there. Other destinations considered by those intending to leave were Australia and Fiji, with one doctor heading for the United States of America, believing there would be better job opportunities for postgraduates there.

The fact that so many doctors were choosing to leave, and to destinations determined by chain migration, presents a somewhat bleak forecast for the future. As people continue to join families overseas (particularly in New Zealand), it can reasonably be assumed that (if immigration laws remain the same) increased numbers of people will leave Samoa and settle in New Zealand. Further studies may be needed to examine the possibilities of changes to the current immigration laws in order to limit the number of people leaving or, alternatively, ways to encourage those professionals who have left to return to Samoa, and hopefully contribute to a chain of return migration to the home country. It may also be of some relevance that, of the five doctors who had no desire to leave Samoa now or in the future, two of them were educated within Samoa and had never had any reason to leave the country. Although no conclusions can be drawn from this evidence alone, it does suggest that it is more likely that medical staff can be retained by educating them solely within their home country.

All of the doctors in the survey were employed on a full-time basis with several working seven days a week and often being on call 24 hours a day. Fortnightly salaries ranged from T$ 580 – T$ 1500, with an approximate average of T$ 835. Over half received regular pay increases, sick pay, pension provision and ongoing training of some description, with a quarter having received some type of housing allowance at some point. The doctors in Samoa appeared to be happy with their choice of career and enjoyed helping people (two specifically listed being able to help Samoan people as being important). Other positive points included the work being interesting (listed by a third of all respondents) and the chance to meet people. Four were happy with the pay and the fact that there were overtime benefits. Interestingly, a further four doctors complained that the pay was too low; however, given the large disparity between salaries, that would seem to be a reasonable outcome. Four doctors were concerned with the heavy workload and almost half felt that the hours that they worked were too long and the time spent on call was unreasonable. All were happy to remain working as doctors, with only one wishing to change from his current position to work as a field officer in the hope that this would be less stressful than his current position.

The evidence suggests that doctors in Samoa are happy with their choice of career but due to long working hours, overburdened schedules and the number of relatives and close friends who are moving overseas, they are unlikely to keep their skills within Samoa for very long. The historic pattern of skilled emigration is likely to continue.

4.3.2 Nurses

The situation among Samoan nurses was somewhat more positive in terms of emigration with only five out of the total of 34 stating definite intention to leave the country. Again, most were destined for New Zealand to join family members. Moreover, less than half the nurses had thought about working overseas at some point in the future, and most of those were drawn by the opportunity to earn more money and increase their own and their children's education, although better medical services and better opportunities for career progression were also considered important. Generally though, the nurses had strong ties to their homeland and often felt obliged to remain because of family ties: "As a Samoan I am responsible for looking after my mother to get more blessings for me and my children." The way of life in Samoa was more important to many than the chance to earn more money abroad with most considering the freedom in Samoa, the low cost of living and low level of crime good reasons to remain. One 67-year-old near retiree declared, "There's no place like Samoa."

Only nine of the 34 nurses had lived abroad for any period of time. Seven had been to New Zealand for study or to visit family, one had been to Japan on a government sponsored training programme and one had travelled to Fiji with her husband on a church scholarship. Seven of the nine were happy to return to Samoa. They tended to have large families in Samoa and were happy to return to nursing and share their newly acquired skills. The two who were not happy had spent time in New Zealand and found the low pay and staff shortages in Samoa hard to cope with. One explained that she and her husband had lots of family occasions to pay for on their return but were now not earning enough money to be able to afford the extra outgoings. Once again, overseas expertise is a critical influence on dissatisfaction and potential future migration.

Wages for nurses in Samoa remain low, averaging just T$ 340 a fortnight. Although income was only important to four nurses when deciding on their choice of career, 18 were unhappy about the level of pay, particularly in light of their heavy workload and the staff shortages that they suffered. The lack of equipment and facilities was also a common cause for complaint, with several concerned about the level of care of patients due to poor facilities. Six mentioned having problems with demanding and complaining patients and it may be that this was one outcome of staff and equipment shortages.

When it came to the positive aspects of their work, the nurses in Samoa tended to display a high level of altruism, with 23 enjoying being able to help people and 17 valuing the opportunity to competently care for their families. Indeed, family was the main reason for nurses entering their profession, with 29 having considered it important for them to gain nursing training in order to care for members of their families. One explained, "As an eldest I was responsible for the health of my family." Another said, "My dad has got heart disease so they asked me to be a nurse so that I can care for him." Given that most of the nurses in the survey had large families in Samoa, and had entered nursing at least in part in order to care for those families, this could be one explanation for them remaining in Samoa when the wages were often inadequate. In a country where family responsibility is considered important, it is unlikely that a nurse would migrate abroad if she had parents or other family members to care for. Altruism seems to be more important for many than monetary rewards, with one nurse even rejecting a better job offer because it would limit her services to those who could afford it: "The MedCen (private hospital) wanted me but I refused it because I know only a few people can afford to come there thus my service too will be limited."

Of the 34 nurses in this sample, the majority were married women with children and settled families in Samoa. The lack of nurses over their mid-30s (only 12 out of 34 were over 40) suggests that there may be a substantial number of nurses leaving the country in their late 30s or early 40s. The nurses within this sample were mostly happy in the home country and content to remain, at least at the present time, but there was no data on how many had already left.

4.4 TONGA

Tonga is a Polynesian state with a population of just under 100 000. Almost as many ethnic Tongans live overseas, mainly in New Zealand, the United States of America and Australia. As in Samoa, the population has not grown for 20 years, as migration balances natural increase. The economy of Tonga has grown steadily in recent years, with agriculture and fisheries being one of the largest sectors. Imports are substantially greater in value than exports, with the difference in value being made up from remittances and aid.

Because of the distribution of Tonga's population over some 40 populated islands, Tonga's health system is more complex and decentralized than in most PICs, with three regional hospitals. However, since about 70% of the country's population now live on the main island of Tongatapu, the central Vaiola hospital plays a crucial role in health delivery. A small private sector meets the needs of some expatriates and those who are willing to pay in order to avoid hospital queues. Medical officers are trained overseas, usually in Papua New Guinea, Fiji or New Zealand, while the training of health officers and nurses takes place locally.

There has been very substantial emigration of medical officers "who have sought and taken positions overseas where better terms and conditions of service are offered", yet despite this migration, almost all posts are occupied by Tongans (World Bank, 1994: 226). Even in the earlier years of emigration, between 1950 and 1975, migration tended to be of the relatively skilled. Typical occupations "for men were the practice of medicine, teaching, administration, trader and the Christian Ministry, with nursing and teaching favoured for women" (Cowling, 1990: 198). While emigration subsequently increased in number and diversified, the skilled component remained important. By the mid-1990s, there was concern that difficulties would arise if numbers under training were not maintained, or the extent of emigration increased, since a significant number of doctors were due to retire in the 1990s.

A survey undertaken in 1995 revealed that 14 doctors had been lost to the health system in the previous 10-year period. One had retired, and at least eight of the others had moved overseas. By then, some five doctors were working in Australia, three were in New Zealand, two in Fiji, one in Samoa and two were unemployed in the United States of America. Several had failed to return from overseas training and had been dismissed from the medical service (Wolfgramm, 1995). While there were suggestions that the primary cause of emigration was economic, and primarily related to salary levels, family reasons – including the location and interests of spouses and other extended family members – were highly influential. A subsequent note has suggested, in the case of Tongan doctors working in Australia, that the key influences were not only starting salaries (since it was argued to be unfair for doctors to start on similar salaries to others such as accountants, whose training was much shorter), but also the unavailability of adequate medical equipment in Tongan hospitals, which made work more risky and resulted in blame being attached to the doctors for inadequate performance (Fisi'iahi, 2001).

At least in the early 1990s, there were few concerns over the emigration of nurses to the extent that the School of Nursing had reduced the intake into first year courses. Only eight new students were taken in 1992, compared with 39 in 1989. Continued reduced numbers would threaten the viability of the school and create concern over staff numbers. Within the nursing profession, there was concern that the career and incentive structure encouraged nurses to enter midwifery and thus remain in hospitals rather than enter general nursing, and that this was therefore at the expense of the rural sector. This situation was hedged with uncertainty since an "important element which has permeated nurse training options in Tonga has been whether the training will be acceptable in New Zealand and Australia rather than [meet] the real needs in Tonga and the Pacific"(World Bank, 1994: 227). Raising training levels to meet overseas requirements had resulted in a situation where it was relatively easy for Tongan nurses to acquire overseas employment, and were thus able to migrate with relative ease.

By the late 1990s, the nurse migration situation had significantly changed. The new training regime had indeed encouraged migration. It is said that as many as 25 nurses emigrated from Tonga in one year, 1998-99 (Rotem and Bailey, 1999: 18). It is worth quoting from the most recent assessment of Tonga's health workforce situation to note the perceived gravity of the situation as seen from within the country:

> Issues relating to staff morale, staff productivity and staff attrition rates are clearly recognized as problematic areas for the ministry. Anecdotal evidence suggests that staff morale has been very low. The reasons are felt to be multi-factorial; however, issues relating to human resource management have been indicated as significant. Poor punctuality and high absence rates from some employees are a source of considerable frustration and irritation to many staff. ... It is felt that there is a disparity of staff deployment across the system. While there are definite areas with staff shortages and a lack of adequately trained staff, it is also believed that there are [sic] considerable overstaffing in some areas, under-utilisation of other staff and recruitment of staff without referral to workload indicators. Another significant area of concern is the high level of professional staff attrition rates. This has long been an issue with respect to medical staff, but is also becoming a major problem for nursing staff and other allied health and technical workers. Low financial remuneration is cited as one of the key reasons for the staff attrition rates but it is also believed that there are other reasons relating to workforce management and communication that contribute to the high attrition rates. Lack of any career development may also be a contributing factor. ... The maintenance of an appropriate skill base within the health system is one of the greatest challenges facing the Ministry currently (Tonga Ministry of Health, 2000: 44).

At that time, some 80 of the intended health workforce of 860 were un-established, and the Ministry saw little prospect of the situation changing in the immediate future. There, as elsewhere, shortages were mainly in the most skilled categories and the impact of these shortages was exacerbated by the prolonged absence of people undertaking training overseas (not all of whom would necessarily return) and the intermittent shorter absences of staff on short courses overseas, conferences and so on (Dewdney, 2000). Labour shortages were most acute outside the main island, especially on the more remote islands, since "no-one wants to go to the Niuas" (Maron, personal communication, 2001). Certainly the workforce situation has not improved in the past decade.

The attrition rate for nurses particularly has created concern as an estimated 10% of all nurses consider emigration in any one year (though the number who actually resign is relatively small, i.e. about 5% of the workforce in a year). Most resign relatively early in their potential working life and it is said that most of those resign to emigrate and that those who are most likely to emigrate are those who have completed courses leading to formal qualifications (such as degrees in nursing) overseas (Dewdney, 2000). Even those who go on short-term overseas training courses are often frustrated by the difficulties in implementing changes on their return, or using newly acquired ideas and skills, to the extent that they often seek to move away (Maron, personal communication, 2001). In other words, within the nursing sector, as within the health profession as a whole, it is the more skilled nurses with overseas experience who appear to be more likely to migrate.

It is not only the attrition of the workforce that is of concern, despite a 20% increase in public service salaries in 2000-01. Although the national health budget is second only to that of education, these funds are grossly inadequate to enable hospitals to provide patients with even the most basic standards (Harkness, 2001: 37). Because of the inadequacy of local hospitals, budget provision exists for transfers and referrals overseas, but only for public servants and members of parliament. This has contributed to enormous frustration with the health system.

A recent study of return migration to one village in Tonga has shown that it is not merely 'failures' and 'retirees' who return, and that many Tongan professionals do return and use their skills, including health skills, within the country. It has also demonstrated the diversity of reasons for migration, and for return migration.

> Accompanying her husband and children, Kaloni migrated to Australia, taking leave from her nursing position within the Tongan Ministry of Health. Her late husband's services were required as a choirmaster for the Tongan Church in Ashfield, Sydney, and as he was not earning very much income and working little, Kaloni completed her nursing registration in Australia so that she could work. Thus she became the breadwinner for her family, working for a health company agency as a locum nurse in hostels, hospitals and nursing homes throughout Sydney, working mainly in palliative care. As a nurse, Kaloni found it easy to support her family, despite working very hard and very long hours, often volunteering to do double shifts. Kaloni also wanted her children to be educated in Australia, and she feels that they have now benefited from their experiences there, particularly from learning English. Kaloni enjoyed her time in Sydney – 'I look forward to going back. I like Sydney. I got enough money... very easy to find a job [as a nurse]'. Maintaining her Tongan identity in Australia was not a problem for Kaloni and her family as they had close contact with other Tongans and attended Tongan church services. Kaloni also made her children and the family speak Tongan at home and English at school/work in order to maintain their Tongan language knowledge, particularly for her children's sake (Maron 2001: 54).

After many years away, Kaloni returned to work in the Tongan health care system, mainly because her husband was ageing and her close family was in Tonga.

Not all movement away from Tonga is of long duration, as in the case of Mele, who worked temporarily in the United States of America.

> A Senior Staff Nurse at Vaiola Hospital, Mele took six months leave in the USA, during which she visited friends and relatives and did relief work in housekeeping and palliative care for her relatives there. In carrying out some relief work, Mele was able to earn a little extra income to complement the amount earned from her role as a nurse in Tonga. After six months in the USA, Mele decided to return to Tonga, mainly because her husband and mother are residing in Tonga, but also because of her nursing position within the Ministry of Health (Maron 2001: 46).

The existence of senior employment, and the presence of immediate kin, largely ensured that superior incomes in the United States of America would not lead to long-term emigration. Scholarship holders too are likely to return, at least in the first instance.

> Due to the lack of tertiary institutions providing medical training in Tonga, Amanaki migrated to Papua New Guinea to study for a Bachelor of Dental Surgery through being awarded an AusAID scholarship to study at the University of Papua New Guinea. He recently migrated to Australia for a five-year period with his family as he was awarded a World Health Organization (WHO) scholarship to undertake postgraduate study there. His wife, Toakase, also chose to enrol in tertiary education in medicine at Fiji's School of Medicine through receiving a Tongan government scholarship. Similarly to her husband, Toakase also received an AusAID (Australian Agency for International Development) scholarship to pursue a Masters in Paediatric Health at the University of New South Wales, Sydney, Australia, allowing her to migrate to Australia with her husband and children between 1995 and 2000 (Maron, 2001: 51).

Each of these diverse examples emphasize that in a variety of contexts, and for different reasons, SHPs return to Tonga, and use their skills for the benefit of national development. Migrants are never entirely lost to the nation.

4.4.1 Nurses

Data from the study indicate that there may still be serious problems concerning migration of nurses from Tonga. From a relatively settled sample of 30 nurses, mostly in their 20s to 40s with spouses, children and large families in Tonga, 15 were planning to migrate at some stage over the next few years. Even if only about half of these nurses eventually leave, the loss represents a large proportion of this sample and, if the group is representative of the wider population, it is indicative of very a serious situation.

There seemed, however, to be no connection between previous overseas experience and the desire to migrate. Eleven nurses had lived abroad at some stage (mostly for study, short working holidays and family visits) and all of them felt that they had made the right decision in returning. Several of them missed Tonga once they had left ("missed Tongan customs", "more comfortable pace of life in Tonga") and several who had studied abroad have gone with the express intention of gaining knowledge in order to help their own people and were glad to return to put their new skills into practice. More than half of these return migrants intended to remain in Tonga.

Most of the 15 people intending to move overseas were intending to live in New Zealand and Australia. Several had no previous experience of these countries but made their decisions based on the assumption that they would have better employment and study opportunities there. Many had family bases abroad and felt comfortable moving to New Zealand because of the Pacific island communities there that would be familiar with their customs and culture, and would enable ease of integration.

One nurse had expected promotion and a pay rise on return from completing an overseas course, but found that she was not entitled as her course was not a Tongan government scholarship. Other than this, complaints regarding low pay were few (although the average full-time fortnightly wage averaged just T$ 310). This could be explained by the fact that 28 of the 30 nurses had entered the profession primarily to help and care for their families. Income was a consideration for very few when deciding on their future career. Greater concerns were voiced regarding perceptions of bad management practice, including the allocation of promotions and a feeling that nurses' suggestions were not considered.

Nurses in Tonga appeared to have moved between hospitals, clinics and departments more than was usually the case for their counterparts in the other PICs. Many had worked in rotational positions in both urban and rural clinics and three had left nursing in order to work as nursing tutors and share their experience with others. Given their varied experience, these nurses would be a particular loss if they decided to take their skills overseas. Apart from the ability to work with people and help patients, several nurses enjoyed the opportunities to work in specific departments and specialize in certain areas (most notably obstetrics and theatre). It would be worth gaining further information to determine whether more staff could be retained if given the support and opportunity to specialize in various areas and what those areas might be. Certainly the evidence suggests that those nurses given flexibility, in training and practice, and therefore greater job satisfaction, were less likely to wish to migrate.

4.4.2 Doctors

At first, the situation with Tongan doctors appeared similar, with 10 of the 20 interviewed stating their intention to migrate from Tonga. However, only one of these had actually made plans to find employment overseas, using academic contacts in New Zealand where he had worked in the past. Frustrated with inefficiencies and lack of training opportunities in Tonga, he planned to leave by the end of the year. Of the remaining nine stating an intention to leave, two were leaving on temporary scholarships for further training, one intended to leave by 2002 but had not yet planned employment overseas, one intended to follow his cousin to Australia but had no set timeframe for the move, and of the five intending to join families in New Zealand, three did not intend leaving for another 2–3 years and the remaining two in the next 10 years. Few were therefore likely to leave in the short term.

The doctors in this survey included 11 males and 9 females with ages evenly spread from early 20s to late 50s. Fourteen were married, 13 with children, and only one lived alone. Most had studied abroad as well as at home, the most common study destination being Fiji followed by New Zealand, Australia and Papua New Guinea. The availability of scholarships had been an important influence in the decision to study medicine for almost half of the group, with family support and the desire for prestige and status also relevant factors.

Of the 15 who had lived abroad previously, most have gone to further their education, although a few had also done some amount of work overseas. One doctor had worked in New Zealand for extra income but had been working to save enough to build a house on Tonga and returned when he had earned a sufficient amount. Most were happy with their decision to return, reuniting with family, preferring a comfortable life in Tonga and contributing to their country's health system. Problems with returning from overseas included adjusting to lower wages and, according to two respondents, finding accommodation near to their place of work.

Of the 17 doctors who expressed some wish to work overseas (although the majority of these chose to remain within Tonga), the main reasons centred around a desire for better educational opportunities for themselves and their children, better career opportunities and the chance to gain overseas experience and travel. Interestingly, only four people listed the chance to earn a better income as a priority. Of the 10 who claimed to be moving overseas, all chose New Zealand and Australia as their preferred destinations on the basis that they had family there, both countries are relatively close to Tonga and have large existing Tongan populations. If income was the main priority for migration, then presumably more doctors would consider moving to countries like the United States of America where earning potential is undoubtedly higher.

The fortnightly salary for Tongan doctors in the survey ranged from T$ 546 – T$ 900, averaging T$ 692. Several worked seven days a week, and 14- to 16-hour days were not uncommon. Despite this, most doctors reported being fairly happy with their jobs, although a quarter complained of lack of facilities, medicines and staff, seven had difficulties with perceived inefficiencies within the administration and bureaucracy of the Ministry of Health, four were unhappy with the low wages and a further two experienced frustrations arising from cross cultural medical issues, particularly with older patients relying on traditional medicines.

4.4.3 Australia

Tongan migration to Australia began in the 1970s, partly due to downturns in the New Zealand economy. Tongans had a greater incentive to migrate to Australia, unlike most other Polynesians, since they found it relatively difficult to establish permanence in New Zealand, and their numbers were increasing particularly rapidly in the 1980s. By the end of the century, there were at least 10 000 Tongans in Sydney, some of whom were illegal over-stayers, and most lived in the Sydney metropolitan area. SHPs have been part of this migration and during 2000, 20 of these were interviewed in Sydney (Fusitu'a, 2000). Seventeen of these were female, all of who have been and usually were still engaged in nursing. One male had become a taxi driver and one female had become an interpreter (though working within a public hospital). The majority had come during the 1980s and all have been in Australia for at least a decade; hence most were in their 40s and 50s, though only one had retired.

Most have chosen to become nurses because it was one of very few professions that women could enter in Tonga and it offered considerable freedom in an otherwise highly regulated society (it was necessary to move out of home and in to the Nurses College). It also offered pay while training and some degree of job security. For several of those in Australia that freedom extended overseas. Nursing, as one said, was "a way of leaving the country." Another explained, "I never forget one of the teachers at home saying to us, 'You know, if you work in another job, like teaching... it's really hard to get a job. But if you do nursing, wherever you go you can get a job.' So I never forgot that. When I arrived here I just went and asked for a job in a nursing home." Nursing thus provided a variety of opportunities, both within Tonga and overseas, that had little to do with nursing itself. Indeed, several saw nursing as offering little prestige. However, most saw their entry into nursing as a means to help others, a perception that they still valued, and indeed helped to define who they were.

The decision to do nursing, or for the men to train in the health professions, was not necessarily their own. Seven believed it was their own choice, seven more said it was definitely not their own choice and the remainder saw it as being a matter of what alternatives were available. One doctor followed his uncle into the profession, a move that was expected of him. Another moved into nursing because her family sought a member in every profession. Indeed, several similar examples demonstrate that the notion of a 'transnational corporation of kin', spreading family resources across countries, can also be seen in terms of spreading family resources through professions (Fusitu'a, 2000). Others moved into nursing for the diverse opportunities it offered, mainly related to some degree of upward social mobility, and the independence and the education were valuable acquisitions. Again, the nature of nursing itself seems not to have influenced decisions to enter the profession.

Those who had practised nursing before coming to Australia described the situation as, in the words of one, being "like in the dark ages". Despite being appreciated by patients, they were frustrated by limited resources. Some worked in remote hospitals without electricity, and for many, access to the basic instruments was sometimes lacking. However, this group had long been established in Sydney.

Most had migrated to Sydney in pursuit of "a better life", for themselves or their children, and nursing provided the means to that end. Several had acquired postgraduate training in Australia (and most expressed the belief that they would not return to Tonga, in part because they would not get jobs commensurate with their new skills and training).

However, rather than seeking great success themselves, the majority focused their efforts on improving the lot of their children or siblings, including those who remained in Tonga. "Those who stressed the fulfillment of their expectations the most were the ones who had achieved the least, professionally, in Australia" (Fusitu'a, 2000: 65). Some perceived that they had become, in their own minds, too free, independent and individualized to return to a structured and hierarchical society like that of Tonga. Many valued nursing because of the flexibility it offered them.

On arrival in Sydney, not all were immediately employed in the health sector, some not having realized that their Tongan qualifications would not be recognized in Australia. Some endured a new training course they had not anticipated. Most had their careers, or the lack of them, altered by economic circumstances, usually related to their spouses' employment, or to such factors as getting married or having children. Despite great diversity within the sample, few had achieved substantial upward mobility within the health system; some were disappointed that they had not achieved greater success but none sought to return to Tonga. Several had children who did not speak Tongan, and would have been unfamiliar and acutely disadvantaged there. Income was not a major issue, and some recognized that salaries in Tonga were adequate to live off. Several stated that the jobs they had now had no equivalent in Tonga, though that might have been "a guiltless way of saying no" (Fusitu'a, 2000: 72), with the implication being that to return and serve was a necessary duty. Others feared the rigidity – and favouritism and nepotism – of the Tongan system. For all of them, the concept of 'home' still "seems to mean Tonga even if they feel they cannot return" (op cit: 73). For many, the simple fact that the majority of their own families now lived in Sydney largely negated that option.

Like Fiji-Indians in Sydney, Tongan migrants were unusual in their relative longevity of residence, and, irrespective of their opinions, the probability that they would not return to Tonga. Nonetheless, despite the fact that several had married non-Tongans and had raised families in Sydney, none had lost touch with 'home' even if return migration was now unlikely. In some respects they remained a resource for Tonga.

4.4.4 New Zealand

A brief study was undertaken of SHPs from Tonga now living in New Zealand. Due to the small sample size and the few similarities between cases, no clear conclusions can be drawn. Therefore, it may be more useful to look at each case individually.

A 38-year-old medical doctor studied in Tonga and then went to New Zealand to pursue further education 20 years ago. She married a New Zealander and never returned to Tonga. Despite the long absence away from her country of origin, she still considered Tonga to be her home and would have liked to return to "give something back to my home country". Unfortunately, the reduced income, poor educational facilities for her children and professional isolation are deterrents enough for her to remain in New Zealand. She earned NZ$ 2500 per fortnight and had no plans to return to Tonga.

A 52-year-old public health physician, educated in Australia and New Zealand, moved out of Tonga in 1980. His wife also worked within the medical field and his three children were born in Tonga, Australia and New Zealand. Although he was planning to leave New Zealand next year, he was leaving to take up a job offer in the United Kingdom, fearing that a return to Tonga would be unsuccessful due to the low income and his fear of discrimination.

A Tongan general practitioner was educated in Australia and moved to New Zealand approximately five years ago in order for his children to receive a better education. He was unable to return to Tonga at the present time due to the high cost of education and lack of a university in Tonga. He did, however, intend to return to Tonga within the next few years as he wished to return to his home country and "help the local situation".

A 76-year-old retiree was educated in New Zealand and Fiji and migrated to New Zealand in 1974 in order to reunite with family. He had lived and worked in the country ever since and had no plans to return, having no remaining family in Tonga.

There exists slightly more data regarding Tongan nurses who have migrated to New Zealand, with 23 nurses questioned for this survey. Overwhelmingly, reasons for leaving Tonga were given as the poor working environment, low pay and lack of education opportunities (for children as well as self). One 50-year-old nurse became so disillusioned with the poor working conditions that she and one of her daughters moved to New Zealand, leaving her husband and other children in Tonga, and had no plans to return. New Zealand was chosen as the migration destination not only because of better pay and conditions, but also because of a chain migration, with the majority of those questioned having existing relatives in New Zealand. As families grow and settle in New Zealand, the likelihood of nurses returning to Tonga decreases.

Only two of the nurses in the survey intended to return to Tonga during their working lifetime. One considered returning to Tonga in order to find a husband (but was not planning to do so in the near future) and the other (who had only recently arrived in New Zealand in the last year) intended to return to help the health service in her own country but was not confident about the outcome, reasoning that lack of funding and resources made change unlikely.

Approximately half the nurses questioned had settled in New Zealand and now considered it home. Several of these still had parents alive in Tonga, but this did not seem to influence their decision and they remained convinced that they would not return. There were those who would consider leaving New Zealand, but future destinations considered were Australia, Canada and the United States of America because of greater opportunities and earning potential.

Others still regarded Tonga as their home (including some of those who had married New Zealanders) and expressed a wish to return, but always after retiring to enjoy the "quiet life". Although many held on to these ideas of homeland and their dreams of a peaceful retirement, few had made any plans to return, and practicalities such as lack of income and other family members wanting to remain in New Zealand meant that this was little more than an abstract idea for most.

Further investigation needs to be carried out to discover the reasons for migrants returning to their home countries and anything that those countries can do to encourage return migration. It is evident that the longer migrants stay away and the more settled they become in their new country, the less likely they are to return. However, neither in New Zealand nor Australia were the migrants entirely lost to Tonga.

4.5 VANUATU

Vanuatu has a rapidly growing population of almost 200 000 scattered over as many as 70 populated islands, which makes equitable health provision difficult. Moreover, rapid population growth has meant that the population per doctor ratio increased by 59% over the last 20 years (while per capita income has fallen over the past five years). The largest town, Port Vila, is on the island of Efate. Vanuatu has a limited economy, based on the production of cash crops, but tourism and a small tax haven are also important.

The Vanuatu health system has traditionally depended on expatriates to a greater extent than most of the other countries in the region, and all those countries included in this survey. As in most other island states, the health system was focused on curative rather than preventative health care. The core of the health system is the 200 or more nurses who are the nucleus of staffing in the five hospitals, alongside about 50 nurse aids. Nurses are trained in Port Vila and attrition of nurses has not been a problem. By contrast, there are some 15 doctors providing medical services in Vanuatu hospitals. However, at the start of the 1990s there were only five ni-Vanuatu doctors in the system "and little prospect for significant localization of the workforce ... unless there is a concerted training effort and salaries are adjusted to become competitive with those in the broader Vanuatu labor market" (World Bank, 1994: 281). This has not happened and Vanuatu remains heavily dependent on expatriate medical officers. In 1999, up to half of the small number of currently practising ni-Vanuatu doctors lived and worked outside Vanuatu, including those in Australia, Tonga and Papua New Guinea (Hassall and Associates International, 1999). With one of the highest doctor to patient ratios in the region, this constitutes a particular problem.

Training of medical officers has also posed a problem. There have been occasions when well-qualified nationals, including those with postgraduate qualifications, have returned to take up specific positions only to be redeployed to duties that are not directly related to the training undertaken. Moreover, a "significant proportion" of ni-Vanuatu doctors who have trained in Papua New Guinea and elsewhere have not returned (World Bank, 1994: 281). The World Bank concluded, "The bonding of students sent both for undergraduate and postgraduate training should be instituted. It may also be possible to reach agreement with neighbours (e.g. Papua New Guinea and Fiji) that they will not recruit ni-Vanuatu doctors trained in these two countries, at least until they have fulfilled the bond" (op cit: 299). Students on scholarships from bilateral donors must return to Vanuatu.

While attrition of nurses has not been a problem in Vanuatu, there was concern at the start of the 1990s that the quality of the nurses was inadequate because of flaws in the training programme. As one senior health bureaucrat pointed out, "What we have here in Vanuatu due to political and economic factors are inexperienced nurses being accelerated through a programme which lacks rigor. Also there are no senior nurses who can act as role models of [primary health care]. The nurses often work in isolation and it is terrifying" (quoted in Kerslake 1993: 66). The critical issue in Vanuatu for the provision of a more adequate health care system is a substantial skills gap (Vanuatu Ministry of Health, 2001) and uneven development, rather than loss of skills through migration.

As in other countries, the remote areas fared worse; in the words of one nurse, who had received special training and upgraded to a more senior position: "Ever since we completed this programme I have had no salary increase, so there is no motivation to improve one's education. In the work setting the support is not there. Transport is poor and I work here by myself and sometimes for months you don't see anyone. We are poorly supervised and poorly supplied with equipment" (quoted in Kerslake, 1993: 72). There is a consistency about descriptions of the situation of support for health workers in rural areas, ranging from the simple lack of contact and moral support to the very real lack of proper support services in terms of supplies, transport and so on. While it is inevitable that rural areas will fare worse than the centre, the reality in large parts of the region is that, as in Samoa (see section 4.3), remote areas and the people who live and work there are out of sight and out of mind. At the very least, a very familiar situation of inadequate housekeeping ensures the continued marginalization of such regions.

Financial constraints during the 1990s have limited the ability of Vanuatu to significantly improve either facilities or salaries within the health system. At the end of the 1990s there was concern that many high-level public service workers were employed on temporary rather than permanent contracts because of bureaucratic inefficiencies within the Public Service Commission and financial constraints associated with the Comprehensive Reform Programme (CRP), part of which involved the downsizing of the public service. This was linked to fears that if the situation did not change "many are likely to seek employment elsewhere – either within the private sector or overseas". This situation then affected 11 government employees in the health sector, for whom similar concerns existed:

> Presently there are some qualified doctors from Vanuatu working overseas – although not for the same reason but due to what one has described as 'poor working conditions'. There is one currently serving in an Australian hospital ... who left in 1997. In Papua New Guinea there is a report that there are two, while in the Federated States of Micronesia there is one. ... There is also a report that a couple of specialized nurses in the field of anaesthesia and intensive care have left for similar reasons (*Trading Post*, 502, 24 November 1999).That article, in a Vanuatu newspaper, was written in response to a letter to the newspaper pointing out that five doctors had gone (though the time period was unspecified) and they were about to be followed by two lawyers. Thus, Vanuatu seems to be moving towards a situation, like that of the other island states, where emigration is now being sought as a response to difficult local circumstances.

An inadequate number of surveys are not yet available from Vanuatu to examine the extent to which concern over 'poor working conditions' remains a problem, and what are the specific working conditions that may pose problems. There was at least some consistency for the two doctors working in Luganville. Both disliked their low salaries, and the difficult and long-duration working conditions, but experienced other forms of job satisfaction, not least the interest and diversity, the sense of achievement and service and some degree of prestige. Both had contemplated overseas migration, for diverse reasons (primarily contact with developments in medicine, continued education and the experience), but both intended to remain because "it's home" and their kin were in Vanuatu. Nonetheless, it is significant that there is now an incipient skill drain from a Melanesian state, which indicates a change in, and a deterioration from, the situation of a decade ago.

4.6 INTENTIONS TO MIGRATE

Statistical analyses of the data (most of which refer to indigenous nurses and doctors presently working within either Fiji or Samoa) yield some generalizations. These focus entirely on some aspects of intention to migrate.

Survey respondents were asked to indicate their intentions to migrate to another country. This section analyses the main factors associated with intention to migrate using a probit regression model where, from the definitions in Table 2, "INTENT" is the dependent variable, which is modelled as a function of the listed independent variables. Means and standard variations are also listed for all variables. There was a total sample of 131 observations from Samoans and Fijians. The overall results of the regression model, summarized in Table 3 demonstrate that the overall goodness of fit for this model is statistically significant at the 1% level, and that most of the independent variables have coefficients with the expected signs and are statistically significant.

Table 2. Intention to migrate model: Descriptive Statistics		
Variable	**Mean** (standard deviation)	**Variable definition**
INTENT	0.3309 (0.4723)	(dependent variable = 1 if answered 'yes')
SAMOA	0.2867 (0.4538)	(country of residence, Samoa = 1)
NURSE	0.7343 (0.4433)	(occupation, nurse = 1)
INCOME	0.0441 (0.0320)	(fortnightly income in A$'000s)
HOUSE	0.6126 (0.4887)	(home ownership = 1 if 'yes')
PLMX	17.2324 (11.7700)	(potential labour market experience = years since graduation)
EXMIG	0.3406 (0.4756)	(previous migration = 1 if 'yes')
YRSAWAY	2.1399 (4.2981)	(number of years lived abroad)
HOMPAR	0.6084 (0.4898)	(parents' residence = 1 if none abroad)
APART	0.1329 (0.3406)	(married but living in different countries)

Country of residence (SAMOA) is significant at the 5% level and shows that if a respondent is from Samoa, then he or she is 21% less likely to be intending to migrate, controlling for all other factors. All other things being equal, this indicates that Samoans are less likely to migrate than their Fijian counterparts. The results also show that there is no significant difference between doctors and nurses in terms of likelihood of migrating once all other factors are taken into account, although the negative sign of the coefficient for NURSE suggests a possible, albeit weak tendency for doctors to be slightly more likely to migrate than nurses.

Income is a significant factor, though only at the 10% level, and the coefficient for the marginal effect suggests a very weak negative relationship between income level and likelihood of migrating in the future. In other words, variation in income within the respondent's country does not appear to matter much,

Table 3 Probit Regression Model Results
(Dependent variable is INTENT; n=131)

Variable	Coefficient	Standard error	Marginal effect
Constant	0.6722	0.7001	0.2099
SAMOA	-0.7789	0.3354**	0.2760
NURSE	-0.1724	0.5146	0.0487
INCOME	-0.0012	0.0007*	0.3771
HOUSE	-0.6859	0.2997**	0.2414
PLMX	0.0819	0.0444*	0.0287
PLMX2	-0.0020	0.9825**	0.0007
EXMIG	-0.4428	0.4003	0.1474
YRSAWAY	0.1483	0.0619**	0.0561
HOMPAR	-0.7145	0.3186**	0.2429
APART	-0.6736	0.4120*	0.2408

Log likelihood function -68.8017
Restricted log likelihood -83.6125
Chi-squared 29.6217***
Degrees of freedom 10

Notes: *** indicates significant at 1% level; **indicates significant at 5% level; * indicates significant at 10% level.

though the higher the income the lower the likelihood of migration. It would still be necessary to investigate the extent to which income differentials between the respondents' country of residence and intended or anticipated destination are important (but that would require subsequent research). Previous general studies of the migration of skilled workers from Fiji to New Zealand (Gani and Ward, 1995; Gani, 1998) have shown that income differentials, alongside political instability, are key factors, so it would be probable that a similar result would occur for what amounts to a subgroup of this population

Home ownership (HOUSE) does appear, however, to be a significant factor, and is statistically significant at the 5% level. Respondents who own a home are 24% less likely to be intending to migrate, controlling for all other factors. This conclusion needs to be interpreted with caution for it could, on the one hand, indicate that respondents who have accumulated sufficient savings to purchase their own home are less attracted to migrate, or it could mean that because they have decided not to move abroad they have decided to purchase a home. The direction of causality is not immediately apparent from this preliminary statistical analysis.

It also seems that the longer the respondent has been in the labour force, the more likely it is that he or she is intending to migrate. There is a statistically significant (at the 5% level), non-linear (quadratic) relationship between years in the labour force and probability of intending to migrate. Each year in the labour force increases this probability by about 3%, but the negative coefficient on the quadratic term indicates that this decreases over time. In other words, the older more experienced respondents are more likely to be planning to migrate, controlling for all other factors.

Despite some ambiguities, the results also show that the respondents' previous migration experiences could be significant in terms of future migration intentions. On the one hand, is does not appear to matter strongly whether or not the respondent has spent some time abroad previously; the variable EXMIG is not statistically significant, and its coefficient is negative, suggesting that, if anything, those who have had a spell abroad are less likely to be intending to migrate again. On the other hand, the longer the respondent has spent abroad the more likely she or he is to be intending to migrate again. The variable YRSAWAY is statistically significant at the 5% level and the coefficient for the marginal effect shows that for every year spent abroad the respondent is 5% more likely to be intending to migrate again.

Finally, the country of residence of the respondents' spouses and parents was also found to be an important determinant of the decision to migrate. The number of parents overseas was the single most important correlate of propensity to migrate. If the respondent had at least one parent-in-law residing in the same country and had no parent or in-law residing overseas, then he or she was less likely to be intending to migrate. The variable HOMPAR is statistically significant at the 5% level and the marginal effect indicates that if this condition held, the respondent was 24% less likely to be intending to migrate, holding all other variables constant.

Where the respondent's spouse was residing in a different country (APART), the respondent was less likely to be intending to migrate. In other words, if the respondent had not already accompanied her or his spouse abroad, she or he was less likely to be intending to migrate than others (although it should be noted that this variable was statistically significant only at the 10% level). This is a remarkable conclusion, which, if valid on a larger scale, has clear implications for a deeper understanding of the 'transnational corporation of kin', with human resources divided across countries.

In conclusion, the findings from this regression analysis suggest that while it is possible to account for much of the variation between respondents in terms of their intention to migrate, it would appear that non-economic, family and demographic factors are equally if not more important than economic factors. However, the issue of relative income and other job-related factors between the respondents' countries of residence and intended countries needs to be explored further. It is highly likely that these significant differences have a clear bearing on migration, but their influence is strongly modified by social and demographic factors. This is very much what the qualitative data also suggest.

4.7 TRAINEES

A short survey was undertaken of students from PICs presently enrolled in health training courses within the University of Sydney. Though the present sample (of just nine people) is too small to reach any clear conclusions, some generalities were of interest. First, almost all the students stated that they had entered the health profession for some combination of altruistic, family and career reasons; several had parents or other relatives who had encouraged this choice of career. Second, almost half the sample were aged 38 or over, suggesting that – at least in Australia – both men and women were willing to take up careers in health relatively late in life. Third, only one expressed any interest in returning to the PICs – "to put something back into Samoa" – and several had become citizens of Australia. Since four were from Fiji, this had some link to political events there. Indeed one Fiji-Indian described herself as part of a "stolen generation". While most of the students had also lived in Australia prior to entry into the training course, this does indicate that the prospects of return migration are poor.

Those who had experienced part of their childhood in Australia were least likely to wish to return to the Pacific. A 19-year-old Fijian, training to be a nurse, who had come to Australia at the age of 14 with her sister, would only return on holiday. Although Australia evoked "bad memories" (e.g. where her mother died, and father left), employment conditions seemed much better than in the Pacific. After four years of education, she now sought "to give something back to Australia". Others echoed similar themes. Once again location of kin was critically important.

By contrast, the sole respondent who intended to return to the Pacific islands was a 45-year-old Samoan woman, enrolled for a Masters course in midwifery, who had been away from the country since 1976 (eight years in New Zealand and 16 in Australia). While she recognized clear advantages to living in Australia, including having an Australian passport, "access to better jobs", "more freedom of movement" and "superior education opportunities", she continued to experience some conflict in balancing her Samoan culture with Australian culture. That she intended to return (though her intent might not be realized) suggests that return migration is always possible. Significantly, she was the only one in this small sample not originally from Fiji. Migrants, and their skills, may never be entirely lost.

5

DISCUSSION

5.1 STRUCTURAL CONTEXT

An enormous amount of information points to the still growing significance of the international migration of skilled personnel, and there is a widespread assumption that it will continue to increase in volume in the years to come. Thus, at a recent (January 2001) conference of the World Economic Forum, education experts argued that skilled migration will continue to be essential in the United States of America, Europe, Australia and the United Kingdom (and, by extension, other countries such as New Zealand) since the primary and secondary education systems of those countries are not flexible enough to prepare children for the skills needed for the flexible thinking required by the new technologies. This shortage of skilled labour in developed countries constitutes the principal global context for continued international skilled migration.

It is equally evident that there is a continued demand in most metropolitan countries for the international migration of health manpower because jobs in the health sector are seen in many metropolitan states as too demanding and poorly paid. Wages in the health sector in most metropolitan states have fallen behind increases in the cost of living, and for these and other reasons employment in the health sector is no longer perceived as favourably as hitherto. Many developed countries, including Australia and New Zealand, the main destinations of Pacific SHPs, have a shortage of SHPs, especially nurses. This has followed high attrition rates and low recruitment. Attrition has resulted from dislike of shift work, lack of flexibility, poor work conditions and incomes and family responsibilities that have resulted in the choice of a job more suited to particular lifestyles. These are broadly the same reasons that SHPs in the Pacific have withdrawn from health services. In addition, work burdens have increased with the ageing of developed country populations. Low recruitment has followed declining birth rates in developed countries; hence there are fewer younger people, and, more obviously, the recognition that there are now many more diverse employment opportunities for women, and that many of those offer superior wages and working conditions, and attract greater respect. Relative declines in public sector funding have enhanced that perception. Consequently, by the end of 2000 nurses represented one of the three professions most in demand for international migration to Australia (within the skilled migration programme).

The international recruitment of nurses has become increasingly global; where once it was mainly a movement from developing countries to a small number of developed countries, typified by the recruitment of nurses from the Philippines (Mejia et al., 1979; Ball, 1996), it has now extended to become more complex, incorporating these continued movements alongside the movement of nurses between relatively developed countries, for example from South Africa and Finland to the United Kingdom.

The international migration of nurses is both temporary and permanent, attracted not only by higher incomes, but also by a range of diverse factors linked to new education and training experiences, family contacts and simply the desire to travel (Buchan, 1999; Hardill and MacDonald, 2000). As a WHO conference noted at the end of 2000, this migration, alongside problems of recruitment of domestic nurses in several metropolitan countries, has left nursing and midwifery services in "crisis". Migration of SHPs in the Pacific region is a small part of this global flow and, with certain obvious differences, shares many characteristics with it.

It is increasingly clear that certain conclusions can be made on the significance of migration, and in the Pacific region, certain generalities appear evident. First, there remains a shortage of skilled health practitioners in all the countries of the region, even in those with the highest educational levels, and that shortage has had to be remedied by various strategies (including retaining staff after retirement age, and recruiting doctors and other skilled personnel from overseas). Neither of these strategies is entirely successful since a series of well-known costs are attached to them. The evidence suggests that the most serious losses of human health resources have come from the stock of doctors, and probably from the small stocks of such workers as radiographers. The situation is less serious for nurses, which is not to suggest that there is an adequate stock of nurses in the region. Even in countries relatively well supplied with health personnel, the cost of referrals remains considerable and may even be increasing (as the wealthy demand certain standards that are unavailable at home). The cost of maintaining health services is substantial.

Second, the lack of SHPs has contributed to the inadequate delivery of health services, especially in remote areas. Though most of the evidence in support of this is anecdotal, the ramifications are evident in the manner in which life expectancies have failed to increase and may actually be declining. (While Papua New Guinea is not directly part of this study, there is direct evidence there of the decline in the availability of rural health facilities, with negative outcomes, and every reason to assume that similar if less extreme situations exist in various other parts of the Pacific region, especially in the Melanesian states.)

It is evident that throughout the region rural and remote areas are effectively 'out of sight and out of mind' and that those who work and live there are marginalized. Policy decisions rarely favour them and failures of 'housekeeping' limit the effective delivery of goods and services. No countries provide any kind of salary supplement for those who work there, and there is very little other real incentive to work there, other than for a handful of individuals who may originate from these areas. The widespread dissatisfaction revealed in these surveys would almost certainly have been even more evident had the surveys not been almost entirely concentrated in the capital cities.

Third, it is evident that the migration of SHPs remains of considerable significance in the region, and no strategy that has been put in place has resulted in any decline in the incidence of this phenomenon. Indeed, few countries have sought to remedy it directly. Moreover, as the case of Fiji demonstrates all too well, whenever there is a political (or other) crisis of some kind, there is an acceleration in the rate of emigration, especially of those with skills. Even more generally, all the global evidence (specifically from the Caribbean, and more recently in this region, from Australia, New Zealand and Palau) emphasizes that countries are increasingly recruiting from (perhaps even 'poaching' on) each other, rather than addressing the 'more difficult' causes of attrition and shortage, that are linked to inadequate pay and working conditions.

Since there have recently been a series of problems in parts of the region to the extent that the Melanesian arc (between Indonesia and Fiji) has been described as 'an arc of instability', there is some possibility that future economic (and other) crises will make the retention of SHPs in the immediate future at least as difficult as it has been in the past. One response to economic problems in the region has been increased fiscal 'prudence', from the mid-1980s onwards, increasingly at the behest of such agencies as the Asian Development Bank. This has usually led to a reduction in the size of the public service, and a deterioration in the working conditions of those who have remained, that has contributed to an acceleration of emigration.

Fourth, all the evidence from trends in the developed metropolitan countries that fringe the region, which have been the traditional beneficiaries of health migration, is that the growing disdain for public sector employment in those countries, linked to relatively poor wages and salaries, will not discourage migration from the Pacific and may even be a stimulus to it. New Zealand hospitals have actively recruited nurses in Fiji. (Moreover, as is eminently clear from within the Pacific, where relatively affluent island states such as Palau, Nauru and the Marshall Islands have in recent years actively recruited migrant health workers from the poorer states, notably Fiji, there is actually a growing demand for health workers not only in metropolitan states, but also in middle-income states. Thus, Palau has recruited nurses in Fiji).

In other words, without exceptional changes in national policy on both public health and migration in recipient countries, any attempts to slow the migration of SHPs must come from inside the region since they are unlikely to come from outside of it. (There is an unfortunate parallel here with the case of the accelerated greenhouse effect.) For the Pacific region as a whole, the context is one where the migration of skilled individuals is likely to continue to be of at least as much importance in the immediate future as it has been in the immediate past.

5.2 SURVEY

While the structural context favours increased migration, the result of the survey point to similar conclusions. There is little indication that the principal reasons for migration, as expressed by individual SHPs, will not continue to be important in the future. Moreover, these reasons may increase in significance in the future. First, a large proportion of all migrants have moved overseas for the 'experience', in a rather nebulous sense, which may relate to social, economic or a wide variety of personal issues (or, perhaps, an unwillingness to discuss particular difficulties). The nature of that experience, in early adulthood, has eventually led to an initially short-term movement turning into a much longer and more permanent migration move (as evident in the experience of so many of the Tongan nurses in Australia). There is no obvious reason why such experiences should be any less welcome in the future.

Second, movements overseas have often been stimulated and facilitated by the presence of extended family and kin overseas, who have supported migrants and sometimes encouraged them. These overseas numbers have increased rather than declined. Indeed, for some island states, such as the Marshall Islands, new overseas communities are being created where none existed before (Hess et al., 2001). Growing numbers emphasize renewed migration.

Third, while there are elements of skilled migration that make it rather different from more general migration streams, migrants remain part of extended 'transnational corporations of kin' whereby their migration is encouraged (or, at the very least, not discouraged) by the financial needs of those family members who remain in the islands. Although the evidence suggests that SHPs make a rather smaller contribution to the economic wellbeing of those who remain at home, compared with those other unskilled migrants who profess the certainty of return migration, they have certainly not divorced themselves from the needs of those who stay. A part of their income continues to be welcomed by those who remain in the islands.

Fourth, one of the elements that makes skilled migration rather different is the way in which migrants are more likely to stress social, lifestyle goals rather than the more economic and educational goals of poorer and less skilled migrants. This suggests sensitivity to any decline in the harmony of the local social environment apparent in the accelerated migration that has followed political tensions.

Fifth, migrants move in order to access superior wages or salaries, better training opportunities and more desirable working conditions. They also move to improve the lifestyles of their children in terms of access to education. These disparities have never substantially changed, and may even have moved in favour of the metropolitan states because of present economic difficulties in island states, and so have increased the propensity to migrate. While the costs of living are high in metropolitan states, that has always been so and has been no obvious (or at least no increasing) deterrent to emigration from the Pacific. It is abundantly evident that this situation is true in a very wide range of contexts. One global review of nurse migration concluded: "In many countries employers have failed to address long standing deficiencies related to hours of work, salary, continuing education, staffing levels, security, housing and day-care facilities" (Oulton, 1998: 126). Even where nurses (and doctors) remain in place such deficiencies are recognized. However, this has certainly resulted in qualified nurses being unwilling to work, producing what is in some part a pseudo-shortage.

Sixth, in most places, it is clear that nurses do not usually enter the profession for the income, but out of some desire to nurse and thus be of value in the community. However, such feelings do not sustain a career, as they become frustrated by low pay, poor (or biased) promotion prospects, lack of available resources, inappropriate workloads and inefficient support systems, especially in remote areas, and hence leave the health service or emigrate. (It is possible that opposition to immigration might increase in destination countries in the future, but little evidence that this will occur or that it would have a significant impact on skilled migrants.) At the behavioural level, therefore, there is additional support for the notion that the international migration of SHPs will not decline in the future.

Two other elements follow that are significant here. First, there is a very strong social component in decisions concerning migration and non-migration. Although economic factors certainly play a significant part in explaining migration, as part of an almost 'standard set' of criteria involving salaries, facilities, career prospects, satisfaction and prestige, they certainly do not account for it. The presence of close kin and perceptions of family obligations are major influences on migration. Some of these factors may be, to some, as seemingly trivial as whether the Prime Minister in Fiji is a chauvinist, and thus unlikely to recognize the needs of workers in a predominantly female profession (see Section 4.1). Most nurses are female and face particular constraints related to partners' careers and family obligations, which may make remote postings difficult. This may be emphasized by security considerations in remote locations (which were, for example, a factor for Tongan nurses posted to the outlying island group of Ha'apai) and make the link with a career structure more difficult to achieve.

Second, as the experience of Fiji suggests, there are (at the very least) political undercurrents that influence migration, especially where these are linked to ethnicity, and skilled migrants are the most able to respond to tensions through emigration. Each of these factors further suggests that migration will not decline in the future.

As the data on Fiji-Indians in Australia clearly demonstrates, some of the strongest influences on migration have little to do with employment, or specifically the structure of employment in the country of origin, but have much to do with time honoured and universal attempts to improve the welfare and status of families in the long run. In that respect, many have entered the health professions less out of altruism, or a particular scientific interest in medicine, but through a recognition that this might be the means to another end, that of maximizing or at least improving family incomes and welfare. Indeed, that is sometimes why parents have encouraged their children to enter the profession. Employment in the health system thus enables migration rather than being an instigator of it. In turn, this further suggests the continuity of the process of migration and, more importantly, its sometimes somewhat tangential nature to the health care system.

However, it is abundantly evident that a perception of inadequate salaries, and obvious salary differentials between the PICs and metropolitan states (and a few territories, such as American Samoa, within the region) underlie migration moves. Moreover, it is clear from almost every survey that has been done of the migration of SHPs from the 1970s (Mejia et al., 1979) onwards, in every part of the world, that a loosely economic rationale dominates migration. Without superior wages and living standards elsewhere, migration would be very slight.

However, wages and poor working conditions are necessary yet insufficient causes, evident in the fact that nurses, doctors and other skilled workers do stay in the region. Those who stay are often older or, conversely, very recent graduates, with strong local family ties. It is equally evident that those who emigrate are primarily those who have been working for a relatively short time, and that, not surprisingly, the stayers are more senior workers, who obtain good salaries, certain privileges and work in favoured locations. This has two possible interpretations; one is that the migrants are highly likely to leave whatever the situation at home (and the evidence from migrants in Vancouver, Auckland and Sydney is supportive of that); another is that restructuring of career paths and promotion criteria (described by many people in different PICS as combining favouritism with nepotism) would reduce migration rates. Social factors are both causes of migration, constraints to it (especially in terms of family structures) and some impetus to return.

It is equally important to note that there is now a very established pattern of migration from several island states, notably Tonga, Samoa and Fiji (but also from the smaller island states), to the extent that migration is a normal occurrence. In this strengthening culture of migration, SHPs are, like other migrants, part of a 'transnational corporation of kin'. Island governments have not usually sought to intervene in the process of international migration, and are unlikely to do so in the future, partly because of the financial benefits that migration brings. Although, as early as 1984, Fiji did commission a study aimed at devising means to reduce the skill drain (Bartsch, 1984), but nothing came from this. Bonding of students is the only policy directed at encouraging return migration. Direct intervention in migration processes remains unlikely.

There are some minor health benefits from emigration. Thus, doctors and nurses, notably in New Zealand, tend to work in hospitals that are attended by patients from the wider Pacific island migrant community, and the ability of these patients to converse with staff in their own language has proved to be of considerable benefit (Barker, 1993: 223-4). Migrants also point to the new skills they will learn and the probability that they will take these skills back 'home', in due course. The actual extent of return migration is poorly understood, though as the surveys have shown it is of some significance for the health services of the Pacific (though less so in Fiji where few, if any, Fiji-Indians have returned), and more needs to be known about its components and rationale to better address the needs of island nations.

6
CONCLUSIONS

When this survey first began, a Tongan public servant commented, not entirely in jest, that there was little point asking Tongans why they had chosen to return to the country because all would simply say "for God, King and country"! A survey of migrant doctors from Fiji in New Zealand recorded one doctor as saying, "We have lost our patriotism in Fiji. No one person or the Ministry can curb emigration. If there is a sense of belonging to the country, no salary, no attraction will be greater than to serve one's motherland. Many no longer feel that about this motherland, this birthright phenomenon" (quoted in Naidu, 1997: 82). Even allowing for a considerable degree of hyperbole, and the impossibility of quantifying such sentiments, they are indicative of the very powerful attachment to 'home', the strong social ties that link islanders to home and the manner in which the structure of community, whatever that entails at various levels, may influence return migration. They also suggest that the potential for return migration is very far from absent.

Nonetheless, given the extent of disillusion that exists among SHPs with the health system in the island states, which is evident both in the number of strikes or threatened strikes in the health sector in recent years, and the general significance of migration from the island states to the metropolitan fringe, which has now existed for almost half a century, it is in some respects remarkable that the situation is not worse. However, it has certainly reached critical proportions, as in Samoa where 40% of all doctors are beyond retirement age and "personnel shortages make it difficult for staff to take leave and go overseas for training" (World Bank, 1998: 19). There, and more generally, health resources are stretched alarmingly, especially in rural and remote areas, and the cost of referrals is increasing. Moreover, the recent situation in Fiji has demonstrated extremely clearly how deterioration in the wider socioeconomic context, i.e. outside the health sector, can dramatically increase the volume of migration among those who are the most highly skilled, and thus have the most easily transportable skills and the greatest ease of entry to a range of destinations. Political fragility can impose unusual costs in small island states.

In terms of outcomes for the health care systems of the Pacific, these are gloomy conclusions in that they suggest not just that a critical development problem is already in place, but that little is likely to change in the immediate future. Indeed, if the experience of other regions of island states, such as the Caribbean, is at all comparable (and there is every reason to think that it is), then the immediate future may last rather a long time. The World Bank too has concluded in a similar vein: "Doctors, especially specialists, remain scarce, often prone to emigrate or move on (in the case of expatriates), and relatively costly. Few work in rural facilities, where medical assistants and nurses provide some curative services. This situation is likely to persist" (World Bank, 1994: 28). Their ensuing policy recommendations bear repeating, in their advocacy of reducing dependence on doctors and generally scaling down the demands on them:

> This can be done by moving physicians out of administrative positions in health ministries, drawing specialist skills from either the local private sector or from periodic visits from expatriates, and by specifying case work loads, with attendant access arrangements, requiring the full skills of doctors (ibid).

In Fiji at least such attempts have been made, but not entirely successfully. While this strategy would better use the skills of doctors presently in the PICs, it is not evident that this would discourage emigration.

Equally, the World Bank sought a wider role for nurses, in the sense that more should be encouraged to work in rural areas and there should be a greater emphasis on primary health care (World Bank, 1994: 28). Exactly the same conclusions apply to this and the Bank itself has observed, "Recognition of the wider role to be played by the various categories of nurses should then be followed up by recruitment of new staff and related steps" (ibid). The implication is that such a strategy would encourage rather than discourage migration.

The World Bank has also emphasized the need for an adequate career structure so that all SHPs have some reasonable expectation of promotion and superior wages. A clear career structure would make it less obviously a form of banishment or punishment to be sent to rural and remote areas (reminiscent in some places of the old Chinese policy of 'rustification'), but more a means of advancement. However, putting in place such a career structure is a complex process in small states, where human relationships are intricate and personal, and where the good middle management required to implement and monitor such policies is largely absent.

What is evident here is that many of the kinds of strategies that are most appropriate for the development of a more effective health care system in the PICs tend not to be in the particular interests of the present SHPs in the region. Most of these are urban residents, with families who are equally wedded to urban life, and are likely to resist relocation in rural areas or what might be seen as de-skilling towards primary health care alongside the loss of a (perhaps) more comfortable and air-conditioned urban office, ward and/or laboratory and library (along with the attendant and affordable amenities of urban life). Indeed, attempts to encourage I-Kiribati doctors to decentralize have been conspicuous failures (to the extent that, at the start of the 1990s, 11 of the country's 12 doctors worked in the only hospital in urban South Tarawa). In Kiribati, experienced nurses with advanced training are mid-level practitioners; they are called medical assistants (MAs). Since the first class of MA graduates in 1979 until 1999, there have been a total of 46 graduates. The majority of the MAs work in the outer-island health centres. The outer islands may be located across the lagoon from South Tarawa (1.5 hours by boat) or thousands of miles across the Pacific (over three hours by plane). There is one MA per outer-island health centre, with populations ranging from 1000 to 2000 persons. There are also MAs posted to Bairiki Health Centre and South Tarawa.

It has been no less difficult to achieve the decentralization of skilled workers (such as teachers) in developed countries (such as Australia). The unfortunate implications of this, and perhaps one of the reasons for the failure to develop and implement strategies of such kinds, is that they appear more likely to weaken the health system by attacking what might be seen as the privileges of those working in it in the major urban centres and thus stimulate further emigration (or simply attrition from the sector). While the World Bank has emphasized the need for more workers in intermediate, less skilled positions, any health care system requires a certain number of skilled and centrally located individuals.

The development of a more effective and equitable health care system will not easily be able to take advantage of the abilities of some of the existing SHPs, as long as the option of migration exists, as it will. The development of a more effective system will depend on the more appropriate training of future SHPs. That conclusion is scarcely new, and PICs have tried to implement policies that would do exactly that, but none of these policies has been successful as the health care profession remains one that is associated with some combination of good wages and salaries, superior skills and high status.

The World Bank has concluded that "salary scales and career paths need to be developed which encourage individuals to become nurses and medical assistants and remain in service in largely rural assignments" (World Bank, 1994: 30). The evidence from most countries is that remaining in rural areas and having a reasonable salary and a 'career path' are incompatible. There is, unfortunately, no reason to believe that the altruism that this appears to imply is more evident in the Pacific than elsewhere.

The Bank also recommended, "Doctors should be paid at least as well as members of other professions (e.g. lawyers) and may need to be given additional allowances and bonuses, depending on labour market conditions and options for emigration" (World Bank, 1994: 30). Elsewhere they have observed, "There is a need for authorities to develop both supply and demand side policies simultaneously to avoid staffing constraints. In particular there is a need to develop professional cadre salary scales and career paths which are not capped by reference to administrative cadre salary scales and career paths and which take account of the propensity to migrate" (op cit: 324). The complexities of actually doing this are apparent in the case of Samoa (see Section 4.3).

Such directions in favour of more adequate salary scales appear to fly in the face of other recommendations, especially in terms of the achievement of decentralization and primary health care, though there is little doubt that (depending on the extent – unspecified – of allowances and bonuses) this would certainly discourage migration. It would also create a very well paid group of workers, whose existence might be problematic on other grounds, notably in the impact on other public service salaries, not only at the highest levels. This would be a drain on the treasuries of small island states. As the Samoan case indicates, where salaries for doctors in Samoa are approximately a tenth of those in nearby American Samoa, let alone the metropolitan United States of America, most countries would not wish, or be able, to raise salaries to anything approaching a comparable level. While salaries at the upper levels of the medical hierarchy might be somewhat better, putting them close to par with metropolitan salaries is financially impossible.

The growing shortage of SHPs in various states has increasingly resulted in movement within the region, as some states (such as American Samoa) are able to offer better salaries, work conditions – and different experiences – and can thus instigate the regional migration of SHPs. This is evident in the present movement of nurses from Fiji to Palau, and other movements from there to Nauru and the Marshall Islands. There has also been some loss of individuals who, following training elsewhere in the region, have remained in those destinations rather than returning home. The World Bank noted that, in the case of Vanuatu's loss to Fiji and Papua New Guinea, that it "may be possible to reach agreement with [these] neighbours, that they will not recruit ni-Vanuatu doctors trained in those countries, at least until they have fulfilled their bond" (1994: 299). It is a measure of the entrenched nature of the problem of migration that it is becoming of considerable significance within the region. Even more significantly, it is indicative of the task of remedying the problem that, as in this case, the onus is seen to lie, at least in part, with the recipient state as much as with the sending state. That poses complex political questions.

One solution is likely to lie in the direction of creating more places for those who wish to become doctors, even though attrition rates are high and the cost of training is considerable. In Samoa, senior bureaucrats saw the response to the issue, seemingly simplistically, as "train more people". In essence, this is the crux of the response, but it is an expensive response. A solution along these lines is certainly appropriate for nurse training and the World Bank has recognized this situation, emphasizing that numerous small, high-cost training programmes need to be upgraded and rationalized. Five (out of six) of the region's nurse training programmes have fewer than 100 students (and Palau can be added to that) and operate in inadequate facilities with high staff-to-student ratios. Low student numbers reflect a policy of limiting admissions, and high standards reflect the production of graduates with credentials that are marketable in Australia, New Zealand and elsewhere (World Bank, 1994: 30). The Fiji School of Medicine has developed a Primary Practitioner course whose graduates would not be internationally marketable but, as the Bank observed, "such initiatives need to be supported through appropriate actions by universities, medical and professional associations and policy makers in Australia and New Zealand" (ibid), but, above all, by the participants themselves. Currently there is little evidence of this.

The key centre for health training in the region is the Fiji School of Medicine (where most Fijian doctors, and many of those from other PICs, receive their training), but it was experiencing problems early in the 1990s with inadequate resources and limited academic strengths. At that time, the Bank concluded that in order to meet national and regional SHP shortages the FSM, and the associated Fiji School of Nursing, should be upgraded so that a "multi-level, multidiscipline centre should be established – capable of meeting Fiji's and most of the region's needs for highly trained indigenous personnel. To implement this objective, existing health training institutions should be incorporated into one Institute, a centre of excellence ... with consequent economies of scale and more effective utilization of scarce expertise, equipment and materials" (World Bank, 1994: 79). This was then an appropriate objective, one that would have acute parallels with the emergence and growth of the University of the South Pacific based in Fiji.

However, it has subsequently become apparent that a centralized School of Medicine for the region would face the same issues that have affected the University of the South Pacific. During the 1990s, there has been growing regional opposition to the USP, partly through a rise in nationalism (resulting in the establishment of local universities such as the National University of Samoa), partly through concern over standards (hence citizens of the other member states outside Fiji increasingly being given scholarship to go elsewhere) and partly through concern over the political stability of Fiji. Hence, what constitutes a reasonable response to regional needs is likely to be frustrated by political change (and the need for such a comprehensive restructuring to be externally funded). Even after the 1987 coups, as Fiji struggled to maintain its political integrity and deal with economic issues, other Pacific states hesitated to send their medical students to Fiji for training. That situation was replicated in 2000.

This is a particular concern given that one of the most consistent findings of this, and almost every other survey of the migration of skilled workers, is that people who have been trained within their home countries are least likely to migrate. Though there may be a particular kind of selectivity among those who are trained at home (that already predisposes them to remain in-country) this does not challenge the need to provide more appropriate courses within country. However, that is an extremely costly exercise, even though it meets the wishes of many countries to have good tertiary training institutes within their countries.

7
FUTURE DIRECTIONS

There is extraordinary consistency in general explanations of migration. Within and beyond the Pacific these focus on low remuneration, inflexible hours, the lack of continuing educational opportunities, limited training facilities, shortages of supplies and equipment and a poor working environment, especially in rural and remote areas (where health needs are least well served). In island states in developing countries this says much about 'good housekeeping' and bureaucratic mismanagement; in a context where mobility (and emigration) are often the norm, governments have rarely sought to discourage it, relatives are increasingly likely to be overseas and public spending cuts are systemic. However social/demographic variables are of enormous significance. The situation is most serious for doctors, especially young and good ones, and more serious in the smallest states. The emigration rates for nurses are steadily increasing. More parts of the Pacific are now being affected by skilled emigration. Migration is no overspill but a definite loss, with clear negative outcomes that are both financial and medical, limiting progress towards healthy islands and possibly even resulting in a regression in that status.

The following are couched primarily as possible directions rather than clear recommendations:

(1) There is an inadequate database on the attrition rates and mobility of SHPs, which makes human resource development more difficult. Few countries presently adequately (or even at all) monitor the migration of SHPs, though all are aware of the gravity of the situation. It would be valuable for each country to have a short questionnaire that could be given to all those who resign that would focus on the specific reasons for migration. Clearly this would be pointless in the absence of a human resource plan for the health sector.

(2) It cannot be overstressed that in-country education, with locally focused curricula, is more effective than out-of-country education, since it is likely to be more appropriate and cheaper, recipients can be more rapidly integrated into the local work environment and the skills are not so easily transferable. However, it is important that graduates from in-country courses are given equal recognition and status as overseas graduates and have equal opportunity for promotion and in career advancement. In-country graduates are certainly less likely to migrate. Providing adequate education in small states where the annual number of graduates required is small indicates that the next best solution is likely to be education at a regional institution within the Pacific. This has clear implications for the strengthening of regional institutions.

(3) Where SHPs are educated outside the region (notably for further education and specialized training) a system of bonding should be in place (even if it cannot always be operationalized). Specialized training is expensive and most countries rely on external support for such training. A bonding system would increase the chances of return and should the trainee fail to return, the reimbursement of training costs would enable others to be trained.

(4) There must be flexible career structures that enable the probability of promotion for the most talented and committed, and that do not neglect those in rural postings. (In a situation where well over half of all health budgets are absorbed by labour costs, it is impossible for countries to pay 'market' salaries that are comparable with those in metropolitan states; hence it is even more important that a promotion structure be in place. Similarly it is important that good performers be 'rewarded' with access to further training, etc.) and that work conditions be flexible. In the context of Vanuatu, it has been recommended that: "career pathways for nurses and other health professionals be reviewed and career opportunities for staff be investigated fully within the constraints of the existing system so that staff who undergo further training receive recognition and career enhancement where possible and appropriate" (Hassall and Associates International, 1999: 29). This is more generally relevant. These are not new conclusions; hence it would be helpful to examine why similar recommendations along these lines in the past have never been implemented, and why it is so widely believed that 'nepotism' and 'favouritism' are rampant.

(5) The most costly attrition and migration rates are among doctors. If numbers of SHPs are to be increased through new or expanded training programmes, or even merely remain the same, the focus should be on nurses who are less expensive to train, less likely to migrate and more likely to be flexible in activity and location.

(6) The greater probability of nurses remaining in place suggests that most countries would benefit from developing new categories of 'nurse practitioner', who are able to be involved in health assessments, screening, care planning, management and coordination, limited diagnostic and prescribing rights and other similar functions. This would simultaneously improve the status (and perhaps the incomes) of the best nurses, compensate for the loss of doctors and relieve the burden on those doctors who remain.

Over the past 10 years, nurse practitioner education programmes were begun in three countries: Cook Islands (only one cycle due to small numbers and inadequate clinical training resources), Samoa and Fiji.

Most mid-level practitioners work under difficult circumstances, in isolated settings where they are responsible for the primary health care needs of individuals and families. The retention of these professionals in isolated, rural and remotes areas is vitally important to health service delivery, particularly to vulnerable population groups. It will be extremely difficult to retain these effective members of the health service workforce, particularly over long periods of time, without essential and functioning components of the health infrastructure and relevant human resources policies and plans in place. The types of administrative and clinical support required by MLPs practising in rural and remote areas include the following:

- clinical career ladders, supporting career advancement for experience and expertise in clinical practice;

- salary structures commensurate with their competencies, responsibilities, education and experience;

- suitable accommodation and safe working conditions, including essential supplies, medicines and reliable and accessible communication equipment; and

- methods of ensuring adequate clinical supervision, continuing education and professional development.

(7) Nurses who remain within the island health systems tend to be those with local kin and family responsibilities. They tend to be older than those who have migrated. If nurses were recruited rather later than at school-leaving age (for example, in their 30s), from those women who are already settled in terms of local social systems, then the likelihood of migration would probably decline.

(8) It may be useful to examine retirement ages. In Fiji, for example, it would be useful to extend the retirement age to 60 (and not 55) to retain doctors who are still of great value, and to remove the inefficient and costly requirement for doing annual contracts to keep such doctors in place.

(9) Improvements in working conditions (appropriate space, equipment, laboratories, etc.) are essential for undertaking the work, boosting morale and increasing job satisfaction, but, unfortunately, there is no obvious reason to believe that island governments will be more committed to this in the future (or have the resources and skilled middle range bureaucratic labour to implement this) than has existed in the past.

(10) In most countries, part of the problem lies in relatively small numbers entering the health professions. The reasons for this have not yet been clearly identified but may have implications for education in high schools.

(11) Though return migration is limited, it clearly occurs. It would be invaluable for any further phase of this study to focus in detail on this, and develop a clear picture of who are the return migrants and why they have returned. It would be extremely useful to examine this by using focus groups rather than questionnaire surveys. This would enable countries to develop programmes/recruiting drives in metropolitan states that might encourage return migration (since return migrants are likely to be of greater utility to the health care system than more costly expatriates). One programme of the United Nations Development Programme, TOKTEN, sought to encourage the 'transfer of knowledge through expatriate nationals', and this approach may have implications for PICs, though it has yet to be examined.

(12) The particular situation of SHPs in outlying areas needs to be examined in more detail since this is where health needs are less well met (and the cost of meeting them through referrals, etc. is considerable) and where practitioners tend to be overlooked (in this survey as elsewhere). This is likely to demand the development of telemedicine (e-medicine) that will link remote centres to the mainstream, enable greater quality health care and let practitioners there keep abreast of new developments. Indeed, telemedicine has particular potential for the continuing health education of health workers, by enabling them to upgrade skills and access relevant and recent information (and not only in remote areas). It is likely to be some time before it is of use for diagnostic purposes. Increasing the availability of adequate computer facilities is also likely to have a range of benefits, especially in more remote areas. Aid donors (such as AusAID) are presently supporting the extension of distance learning within areas such as health, but (as in Tonga) these opportunities are not proving easy to extend because of inadequate and expensive access to the Internet.

(13) Countries need to consider the possibility of developing some forms of 'twinning'/linkage between national health care systems, and overseas institutions, that would link training in those institutions, with support from them for particular health care problems, on a short or long-term basis, in the event of a sustained shortage of human resources. (A particular model has been proposed for Cook Islands, based on the experience of the small Caribbean state of St. Lucia with short-term volunteers from the United States of America).

(14) Emigration cannot take place without metropolitan states enabling this. There is a need for metropolitan recipient countries (e.g. Australia, New Zealand, United States of America and Canada) to review policies for international migration where these are a serious constraint to the retention of skilled workers in the PICs. (It may also be necessary for some PICs to examine their own recruitment practices where these affect other PICS; this again emphasizes the need for the strengthening of regional institutions so that they produce adequate human resources.) The labour market within metropolitan countries suggests that this is unlikely, yet it is evident that the present structure of attrition and migration could not

take place without a substantial input of development aid (which is presently being 'wasted', at least for the aid recipient countries).

(15) There may be a need for the development of legislation to regulate the role of recruitment contractors (if these are prejudicial to human resource management in PICs). Any existing international recruitment guidelines (such as the proposed Commonwealth Code of Practice for International recruitment of health workers) should be considered as a possible mechanism for reducing any adverse impacts of SHPs migration.

(16) It may be necessary to develop more appropriate mechanisms to regulate the licensing and qualification requirements of immigrant SHPs (though the evidence suggests that, even with some disadvantages, they are making significant contributions

(17) It may be useful to extend this study to look at the situation of other migrant categories (e.g. dentists) where the context may be different from that of medical officers and nurses, and the numbers are so few that even a very small attrition rate is critical (although, at this interim stage, there is no reason to believe that it is different).

REFERENCES

Ahlburg D and Levin M. *The North East Passage: A Study of Pacific Islander Migration to American Samoa and the United States*. NCDS Pacific Research Monograph No.23, ANU, Canberra, 1990.

Azam A. *Motivation of Doctors within the Fiji Civil Service* [MBA dissertation]. Suva, University of the South Pacific, 1996.

Baer L, Gesler W and Konrad T. The wineglass model: tracking the locational histories of health professionals. *Social Science and Medicine*, 2000, 50:317-329.

Ball R. Nation building: the globalization of nursing – the case of the Philippines. *Pilipinas*, 1996, Fall, 27:67-92.

Barker JC. Pacific Islanders in New Zealand Hospitals. In: McCall G and Connell J, eds. *A World Perspective on Pacific Islander Migration*. Sydney, Centre for South Pacific Studies, 1993:209-228.

Bartsch W. *The Skill Drain from Fiji: Situation and Possible Remedies*. Suva, Central Planning Office, 1974.

Bertram I. The MIRAB Model Twelve Years On. *The Contemporary Pacific*, 1999, 11: 105-138.

Bertram I and Watters R. The MIRAB Economy in South Pacific microStates. *Pacific Viewpoint*, 1985, 26:497-520.

Brown, M. Flight of doctors deals body blows to the system. *Sydney Morning Herald*, 2 August 2000.

Brown M. Yet another doctor gives up and packs his bags. *Sydney Morning Herald*, 3 August 2000.

Buchan J and O'May F. Globalisation and Healthcare Labour markets: a Case Study from the United Kingdom. *Human Resources for Health Development Journal*, 1999, 3.

Christensen PM. *Infant Nutrition and Child Health on Tarawa, Kiribati*. Sydney, University of New South Wales, 1995 (Pacific Studies Monograph No. 15).

Cobb-Clark D and Connolly M. A Worldwide Market for Skilled Migrants: Can Australia Compete? *International Migration Review*, 1997, 31:670-693.

Commonwealth Secretariat. *A Future for Small States. Overcoming Vulnerability*. London, Commonwealth Secretariat, 1997.

Cook Islands. *Cook Islands Development Plan 1982-1985*. Rarotonga, 1984.

Connell J. Population Growth and Emigration: Maintaining a Balance. In: Taylor M, ed. *Fiji. Future Imperfect?* Sydney, Allen and Unwin, 1987:14-32.

Connell J. *Sovereignty and Survival. Island MicroStates in the Third World*. Sydney, Department of Geography, University of Sydney, 1988 (Research Monograph, No.3).

Connell J. Health in Papua New Guinea: a decline in development. *Australian Geographical Studies*, 1997, 35:271-293.

Crocombe R. Rural Development, *Pacific Perspective*, 1978, 7(1-2):42-59.

Dever G. Physician Training in Micronesia – the Next Generation [unpublished]. Paper to South Pacific Commission Thirteenth Regional Conference of Permanent Heads of Health Services, Noumea, 1991.

Dever G, Finau S and Hunton R. The Pacific medical education model, *Pacific Health Dialog,* 1997, 4(1):177-190.

Dewdney J. *Kingdom of Tonga National Health Workforce Plan 2001-2020.* Nuku'alofa, Ministry of Health, 2000.

Emery S. *The Samoans of Los Angeles.* Los Angeles, University of Southern California, 1976.

Fatupaito M. American delinquents rehabilitated in Paradise – the inside story. *Talamua,* 19-21 February 1997, 4 (1).

Finau, S. Bureaucracy and the Pacific Health Services. *Journal of Pacific Studies,* 1988, 14:131-134.

Findlay A, Li F, Jowett A, Brown M and Skeldon R. Doctors diagnose their destination: an analysis of the length of employment abroad for Hong Kong doctors. *Environment and Planning A,* 1994, 26:1605-1624.

Findlay A. Skilled transients: the invisible phenomenon? In: Cohen R, ed. *The Cambridge Survey of World Migration.* Cambridge, Cambridge University Press, 1995: 515-522.

Fisi'iahi FV. Labour Migration from Tonga – of more benefit than harm? In: Naidu V, Vasta E and Hawksley C, eds. *Current Trends in the South Pacific Migration.* Wollongong, Asia Pacific Migration Research Network, 2001:41-53 (Working Paper No. 7)

Fusitu'a P. *My Island Homes: Tonga, Migration and Identity* [BA honours thesis]. Sydney, University of Sydney, 2000.

Gani A. Some empirical evidence on the determinants of immigration from Fiji to New Zealand: 1970-1984. *New Zealand Economic Papers,* 1998, 32:57-69.

Gani A. Some dimensions of Fiji's recent emigration. *Pacific Economic Bulletin,* 1999, 15(1):94-103.

Gani A and Ward BD. Migration of professionals from Fiji to New Zealand: a reduced form supply-demand model. *World Development,* 1995, 23:1633-1637.

Gould M and Moon G. Problems of providing health care in British island communities. *Social Science and Medicine,* 2000, 50:1081-1090.

Hamnett M and Connell J. Diagnosis and Cure: the resort to traditional and modern medical practitioners in the North Solomons. *Social Science and Medicine,* 1981, 15B: 489-498.

Han ST. New horizons in health: a perspective for the 21st century. *Pacific Health Dialog,* 1996, 2(1):253-258.

Hardill I and MacDonald S. Skilled international migration: the experience of nurses in the United Kingdom. *Regional Studies,* 2000, 34:681-692.

Harkness L. Recent economic developments in the Kingdom of Tonga. *Pacific Economic Bulletin,* 2001, 16(1):19-43.

Harrison ME. Female physicians in Mexico: migration and mobility in the lifecourse. *Social Science and Medicine,* 1998, 47:455-468.

Hassall and Associates International. *Vanuatu Health Sector Planning and Management Development Report,* Canberra, 1999.

Hess J, Nero K and Burton M. Creating Options: Forming a Marshallese Community in Orange County, California. *The Contemporary Pacific,* 2001, 13:89-121.

Hooker K and Varcoe J. Migration and the Cook Islands. In: Overton J and Scheyvens R, eds. *Strategies for Sustainable Development. Experiences from the Pacific.* Sydney, UNSW Press, 1999:91-99.

Iredale R. Skilled Migration Policies in the Asia-Pacific Region. *International Migration Review,* 2000, 34:882-906.

Ishi T. Class Conflict, the State and Linkage: the International Migration of Nurses from the Philippines. *Berkeley Journal of Sociology,* 1987, 32:281-312.

Kerslake MT. *The Nurse Practitioner in the South Pacific Region* [M.Sc. (PHC) thesis]. Adelaide, Flinders University, 1993.

Koser K and Salt J. The Geography of Highly Skilled International Migration. *International Journal of Population Geography,* 1997, 3:285-303.

Lander H and Miles V. *The Fiji School of Medicine.* Sydney, Centre for South Pacific Studies, 1992.

Lewis ND. More Than Health Services: Health For Pacific Peoples. *Regional Development Dialogue,* 1990, 11(4): 76-96.

Lewis ND and Rapaport M. In a sea of change: health transitions in the Pacific. *Health and Place,* 1995, 1:211-226.

Liki A. *E Tele A'A O Le Tagata. Career Choices of Samoan Professionals within and beyond their Nu'u Moni* [MA thesis]. Suva, University of the South Pacific, 1994.

Liki A. Moving and Rootedness: the paradox of the Brain Drain among Samoan Professionals. *Asia-Pacific Population Journal,* 2001, 16:67-84.

McGrath BB (1999) Swimming from Island to Island: Healing Practice in Tonga, *Medical Anthropology Quarterly,* 13, 483-505.

McKendry R, Wells G, Dale P, Adam O, Buske L, Strachan J and Flor L. Factors influencing the emigration of physicians from Canada to the United States. *Canadian Medical Association Journal,* 1996, 154:171-181.

Macpherson C. The Skills Transfer Debate: Great Promise or Faint Hope for Western Samoa? *New Zealand Population Review,* 1983, 9(2):47-76.

Marcus GE. Power on the extreme periphery: the perspective of Tongan elites in the modern world system. *Pacific Viewpoint,* 1981,22:48-64.

Maron N. *Return to Nukunuku. Identity, Culture and Return Migration to Tonga* [BA Honours Thesis]. The University of Sidney, 2001.

Mejia A, Pizurki H and Royston E. *Physician Migration and Nurse Migration. Analysis and Policy Implications.* Geneva, WHO, 1979.

Mitchell R. Fiji's health system since the coup. In: Prasad S, ed. *Coup and Crisis: Fiji – A Year Later.* Melbourne, Arena, 1988:75-78.

Naidu LK. *Contemporary Professional Emigration from Fiji* [MA thesis]. Suva, University of the South Pacific, 1997.

Oommen TK. India: 'Brain Drain' or Migration of Talent? *International Migration,* 1989, 27:411-422.

Oulton J. International trade and the nursing profession. In: Zarrilli S and Kinnon C, eds. *International trade in health services: a development perspective.* Geneva, UNCTAD and WHO, 1998:125 133.

Parliament of the Commonwealth of Australia. *In the pink or in the red? Inquiry into the provision of health services on Norfolk Island.* Canberra, Joint Standing Committee on the National Capital and External Territories, 2001.

Pollock N and Finau S. Health. In: Rapaport M, ed. *The Pacific Islands. Environment and Society.* Honolulu, Bess Press, 1999:282-295.

Polu L. My Day As A Doctor. *Talamua,* 11-18 December 1999, 6 (11).

Rees TP. Nurses show true meaning of sacrifice. *Samoa Observer,* 27 April 2000.

Ritchie J, Rotem A and Hine B. Healthy Islands: from concept to practice. *Pacific Health Dialog,* 1998, 5:180-186.

Rotem A and Bailey M. Health Personnel Migration within Commonwealth countries in the Pacific region. Sydney, UNSW, 1999.

Rotem A and Dewdney J. *The Health Workforce. South Pacific Island Nations.* Sydney, WHO/UNSW, 1991.

Samuel S and Samo M. Bringing Health Care to the People. *Micronesian Counselor*, 2000, No. 24.

Shankman P. *Migration and Underdevelopment: The Case of Western Samoa.* Boulder, Westview Press, 1976.

Shore B. Introduction. In: Macpherson C, Shore B and Franco R, eds. *New Neighbors...Islanders in Adaptation.* Santa Cruz, Center for South Pacific Studies, 1978.

Taitai T. *Health System Reform in the Western Pacific Region.* Manila, WHO, 1999.

Taylor R. Problems of Health Administration in Small States: Observations from the Pacific. In: Ghai Y, ed. *Public Administration and Management in Small States. Pacific Experiences.* Suva, Commonwealth Secretariat and USP, 1990:60-114.

Taylor R, Lewis ND and Sladden T. Mortality in Pacific Island Countries around 1980: geopolitical, socio-economic, demographic and health service factors. *Australian Journal of Public Health*, 1991, 15:207-221.

Thomason J, Newbrander W and Kolehmainen-Aitken R-L. *Decentralization in a developing country: the experience of Papua New Guinea and its health service.* Canberra, ANU, 1991 (NCDS Pacific Research Monograph, No. 25).

Tonga Ministry of Health. *Tonga's Health 2000.* Nuku'alofa, Ministry of Health, 2000.

United Nations Development Programme. *Sustainable Human Development in Palau.* Suva, UNDP, 1998.

United Nations Development Programme. *Pacific Human Development Report 1999*/ Suva, UNDP, 1999.

Vanuatu Ministry of Health. *2001 Human Resource Development Plan.* Port Vila, Ministry of Health, 2000.

Ward M. *The Role of Investment in the Development of Fiji.* Cambridge, Cambridge University Press, 1971.

de Wenden CW. East-West and North-South brain drain: a comparison of the flows in Western Europe. *Studi Emigrazione*, 1995, 117:90-97.

Workman R, O'Meara C, Craig J, Nagel J, Robbins E and Ballendorf D. *Island Voyagers in New Quests.* Micronesian Area Research Center, University of Guam, 1981.

Wolfgramm S. Comments made by the National Health Development Committee on the Proposed Salary Structure and Interim Salary Revision for the Government Medical Practitioners of the Kingdom of Tonga [mimeo]. Nuku'alofa, Ministry of Health, 1995.

World Bank. *Health Priorities in the World Bank's Pacific Member Countries.* Washington, World Bank, 1994.

World Bank. *Samoa Health Sector Review. Meeting the Challenges of Development.* Washington, World Bank, 1998.

World Health Organization. *Country Health Information Profiles.* Manila, WHO, 1999.

APPENDIX I

SURVEY QUESTIONNAIRE—MIGRANTS
CONFIDENTIAL

2000
WHO MIGRATION STUDY

Undertaken for the World Health Organization
by
Associate Professor John Connell
School of Geosciences
University of Sydney
NSW 2006
Australia0

e-mail: connelljohn@hotmail.com

INTERVIEW SERIAL NUMBER: ☐☐☐

INTERVIEWER NAME: _____ ☐

COUNTRY: _____ ☐

CITY/TOWN: _____ ☐

DATE OF INTERVIEW: _____

Name: _____

Address: _____

Age: _____ ☐

Sex: F ☐ 0   M ☐ 1

Normal place of residence (name of city/town/village) _____ ☐☐☐

Ethnicity _____ ☐☐

Birth Place _____ ☐☐

1. Who lives in your household?

	Relationship to Respondent	Code	Age	Sex	Highest education level	Code (see Q4)	Occupation	Code	Country of birth	Code (see Q39)
1										
2										
3										
4										
5										
6										
7										
8										
9										
10										
11										
12										
13										
14										
15										
16										

2. Your present occupation _____ **Code** ☐☐

   Location/employer _____ ☐☐

EDUCATION

3. Where? _____ **Code** ☐☐ When completed? _____

   What is your highest level of education and qualification obtained (Tick on box only)?

		Code
Primary school	☐	1
Secondary/high school	☐	2
Nursing College	☐	3
Medical School/ University degree	☐	4
Postgraduate degree	☐	5
Other (please specify) _____	☐	6

   Code

   At what type of institution/college did you study? _____ ☐☐
   [University?, Nursing School?, Medical School?]

   When completed? (year) _____

4. Why did you become a nurse/doctor?
   [Tick up to 3 boxes and indicate the **most important,** numbering them "1", "2" and "3")

		Code
income	☐	
enable migration	☐	
family	☐	
prestige/status	☐	
altruism/to do good	☐	
other (specify) _____	☐	

   Did your family want you to become a nurse / doctor?

   Yes ☐   No ☐ ➔ *Go to question 6*   **Code**
   ⬇
   Why? (Give the most important reason only) _____ ☐☐

5. What was your previous employment in the Pacific Islands?
   [Last three jobs only]

   #1:   What? _____ ☐☐
         Where? (Institution, Place) _____ ☐☐
         When (give years)? 19_____ to 19_____

   Why did you leave that job?_____ ☐☐

   #2:   What? _____ ☐☐
         Where? (Institution, Place) _____ ☐☐
         When (give years)? 19_____ to 19_____

   Why did you leave that job?_____ ☐☐

   #3:   What? _____ ☐☐
         Where? (Institution, Place) _____ ☐☐
         When (give years)? 19_____ to 19_____

   Why did you leave that job?_____ ☐☐

6. Since graduating from medical/nursing school, what type of jobs have you had in this country? Specify if employment was in an urban or rural area. (Tick the appropriate boxes)

		Job (1)	Urban (2)	Rural	Code	
a)	resident hospital appointment	☐	☐	☐	01	
b)	private general practice	☐	☐	☐	02	
c)	private general practice/partnership	☐	☐	☐	03	
d)	private specialist practice ☐	☐	☐		04	
e)	private specialist practice/partnership	☐	☐	☐		
f)	government health clinic ☐	☐	☐		05	
g)	government / public service	☐	☐	☐	06	
h)	armed services	☐	☐	☐	07	
i)	teaching and / or research	☐	☐		08	
j)	unemployed ☐	☐	☐		09	
k)	decided to emigrate abroad, directly after graduation ☐	☐	☐		10	
l)	other medical work not mentioned (Please specify below) ☐	☐	☐		11	
	_____				20	
m)	other non-medical work not mentioned (Please specify below)	☐	☐	☐	30	
	_____					

MIGRATION

7. What year did you come to live in this country? _____

8. Are you a citizen of this country? No ☐   Yes ☐ ➔ *Go to question 10*
   ⬇
   What passport do you hold? _____

9. Have you ever lived in another country, for longer than six months besides this one and your 'home country'?

   Yes ☐   No ☐ ➔ *Go to question 11*
   ⬇

Country	Code (see Q39)	How long did you live there (years)?	When? (dates)	Why?	Code	If employed, why did you leave this job?	Code

11. Why did you leave the previous country you were working/living in to come here?
    (Tick as many boxes as you consider relevant but also indicate the 3 most important, numbering them as "1", "2" and "3".

Code	
01	☐ unemployed and seeking work
02	☐ to seek work for the first time
03	☐ unsatisfactory earnings/much better earnings here
04	☐ work conditions or benefits unsatisfactory
05	☐ personal problem with employer or others at work
06	☐ inadequate educational opportunities there, wanted more education for self
07	☐ inadequate educational opportunities there, wanted more education for children
08	☐ inadequate amenities, social activities there
09	☐ to get married, prospective spouse being in this country
10	☐ personal conflicts with family / relatives / friends / community there
11	☐ lack of close relatives, friends in the area
12	☐ to accompany or join spouse to accompany or join other relative
13	☐ to accompany or join friend
14	☐ political problems, felt persecuted or at risk of government persecution
15	☐ a possible opportunity to migrate elsewhere later
16	☐ overseas experience / travel
20	☐ other, (specify)_____

12. Prior to this job had you been to this country before?

    Yes ☐   No ☐ → *Go to question 13.*
    ↓
    When (year/years)?_____
    Why?_____

13. Why did you migrate to this particular country?
    (Tick as many boxes as you consider relevant but also indicate the 3 most important, numbering them "1", "2" and "3")

Code	
01	☐ higher wages, higher income levels here, hoped to get a better job
02	☐ offered better job here before I came
03	☐ transferred by employer
04	☐ good business opportunities here, good place to invest
05	☐ to obtain more education for self
06	☐ to obtain better or more education for children
07	☐ had spouse waiting for me here
08	☐ better prospects for finding a spouse
09	☐ better amenities here
10	☐ better medical and health services here
11	☐ less insecurity in this country
12	☐ fewer environmental problems
13	☐ have friends and relatives here
14	☐ easier to meet migration requirements
15	☐ this is my home country
20	☐ other, specify_____

14. Why did you migrate to that country (eg. Australia, New Zealand) as opposed to other possible destinations, (e.g. USA or Australia or ….)?

Code	
01	☐ higher wages, higher income levels here, hoped to get a better job
02	☐ offered better job here before I came
03	☐ transferred by employer
04	☐ good business opportunities here, good place to invest
05	☐ to obtain more education for self
06	☐ to obtain better or more education for children
07	☐ had spouse waiting for me here
08	☐ better prospects for finding a spouse
09	☐ better amenities here
10	☐ better medical and health services here
11	☐ less insecurity in this country
12	☐ fewer environmental problems
13	☐ have friends and relatives here
14	☐ easier to meet migration requirements
20	☐ other, specify_____

15. Who primarily made the decision for you to move to this country?

Code	
01	☐ Myself
02	☐ Spouse
03	☐ child (ren)
04	☐ parent (s)
05	☐ other relative, specify
10	☐ employer
20	☐ other, specify

Please explain how the decision was made for you to move to this country

_____
_____
_____   ☐☐

16. Before you came here, what were your main sources of information about this country? (Tick as many boxes as you consider relevant but also indicate the 3 most important, numbering them "1", "2" and "3")

Code	
01	☐ relatives, friends already living here
02	☐ relatives, friends living in previous country of residence
03	☐ private employment agencies, labour recruiters from this country
04	☐ government employment agency from this country
05	☐ television
06	☐ radio
07	☐ movies
08	☐ written media: newspapers, magazines, (specify exact source)
09	☐ other, specify_____

Please describe the type of contact you had with the most influential source, (including the first contact or information you remember, frequency of contact, how it affected your views about this country or other countries you may have been thinking about, etc...).

Type of contact	Code	First contact or information	Code	Frequency of contact	Code	How it affected your views about this country or other countries	Code

17. Before you moved to live here, did you have any information specifically about employment/work opportunities?

Yes ☐   No ☐ → *Go to question 18.*

Code	
01	☐ relatives, friends living in this country
02	☐ relatives, friends living in previous country of residence
03	☐ private employment agencies in this country
04	☐ newspaper, radio, tv
05	☐ visited this country earlier
06	☐ labour recruiter, contractor
07	☐ employer
09	☐ other, specify_____

18. What was your marital status when you arrived in this country?

   Single ☐   Married ☐

19. [Nurses only] Before you came to this country did you have any contact with a recruitment agent?

   Yes ☐   No ☐ → *Go to question 20.*
   ↓
   What transpired?_____

20. Did you experience difficulties waiting to migrate to this country?

   Yes ☐   No ☐ → *Go to question 21*
   ↓
   If so, what?_____

EMPLOYMENT

21. When you moved to this country did you have a job waiting for you?   Yes ☐   No ☐

22. Who helped you get a job here?

Code	
01	☐ no one
02	☐ relative
03	☐ friend,
04	☐ employer, business contact, or associate
05	☐ migrant community or ethnic association, specify which
06	☐ trade union
09	☐ other, specify_____

23. Did you have any relatives or friends in this country before you moved to live here?

Yes ☐ No ☐ → *Go to question 24*
↓

Did any of your relatives or friends living in this country help you in any way when you first came here?

Yes ☐ No ☐ → *Go to question 24*
↓

What were the main types of assistance they gave you when you first moved to this country?

Code	
01	☐ obtained visa
02	☐ paid for transportation
03	☐ provided lodging and food
04	☐ provided money/loan
05	☐ provided information about job possibilities
06	☐ helped to find employment/work
07	☐ helped to find house, apartment or other lodging
08	☐ provided full support until I found a job
09	☐ other, specify_____

24. Who paid for you to get to this country?

Code	
01	☐ self
02	☐ relative
03	☐ friend
04	☐ employer, business contact, or associate
05	☐ migrant community
06	☐ ethnic association
07	☐ trade union
08	☐ labour recruiter or contractor
09	☐ other, specify_____

25. Apart from relatives in this country, after you arrived in this country, what was your main means of support?

Code	
01	☐ the job that I already had waiting for me in this country
02	☐ personal savings
03	☐ loan
04	☐ trade union in this country helped
05	☐ relatives in previous country of residence or in home country
06	☐ migrant community, ethnic or migrant association in this country
07	☐ casual jobs in this country
09	☐ other, specify_____

26. How long were you in this country before you started looking for work?

Code	
01	☐ Less than a month
02	☐ Within 6 months
03	☐ Never

27. What were the main methods that you used to seek work after you arrived?

Code	
01	☐ friends, relatives in this country
02	☐ friends, relatives in previous country of residence
03	☐ private employment agency in this country
04	☐ government employment agency in this country
05	☐ I read newspapers and other printed material looking for job openings
06	☐ I asked or visited potential employers
07	☐ I tried to set up business
09	☐ other, specify_____

28. What was your previous employment in this country? [Last three jobs only]

#1: What? _____ ☐☐

Where? (Institution, Place) _____ ☐☐

When (give years)? 19_____ to 19_____

Why did you leave that job?_____ ☐☐

#2: What?_____ ☐☐

Where? (Institution, Place)_____ ☐☐

When (give years)? 19_____ to 19_____

Why did you leave that job?_____ ☐☐

#3: What?_____ ☐☐

Where? (Institution, Place)_____ ☐☐

When (give years)? 19_____ to 19_____

Why did you leave that job?_____ ☐☐

29. Since you were employed here in health related jobs, have you received any on the job training?

   Yes ☐   No ☐ →   *Go to question 30*
   ↓
   What?_____

30. How many days do you work per week? ☐

   Hours per day? ☐☐

31. What is your present income? (per fortnight) ☐☐☐☐☐☐

32. Do you have a regular salary/wage increase?   Yes ☐   No ☐

   Some employers provide their employees with certain benefits, such as a retirement program, health insurance, housing, etc. Do you receive any benefits like these from your current employer?

   Yes ☐   No ☐ →   **Go to question**
   ↓
   What benefits do you receive? (Tick those that apply)

Code		
1	☐	health insurance, medical care, sick leave
2	☐	retirement pension / superannuation
3	☐	unemployment benefits
4	☐	housing
5	☐	training
9	☐	other, specify_____

JOB

33. What do you like most about this job? [Give up to 3 reasons in order of importance]

   1._____

   2._____

   3._____

34. What do you dislike most about this job? [Give up to 3 reasons in order of importance]

   1._____

   2._____

   3._____

35. Would you like a different job?   Yes ☐   No ☐

What?_____

Why? [Give up to 3 reasons in order of importance]

1. _____

2. _____

3. _____

36. Are you trying to get a new job?   Yes ☐   No ☐

37. Is anybody else in this household employed?   Yes ☐   No ☐ → *Go to question 38*

	Relationship to Respondent	Code	Where	Code	Occupation	Code	Income (per fortnight)
1							
2							
3							
4							
5							
6							

Would any of them like to change jobs?   Yes ☐   No ☐ → *Go to question 38*
↓

To what job and where?_____

38. Do you own a house here?   Yes ☐   No ☐ → Do you rent?   Yes ☐ No ☐
↓
Is it paid off?   Yes ☐   No ☐

Do you live with relatives?   No ☐   Yes ☐
↓
Do relatives live with you?   Yes ☐   No ☐

Do you own a telephone?   Yes ☐   No ☐

Do you own a car?   Yes ☐   No ☐

Do you own a house elsewhere?   Yes ☐   No ☐

Do you own land elsewhere?   Yes ☐   No ☐

Do you own a business?   Yes ☐   No ☐ → *Go to question 39*
↓

	Type of business	Code	Where	Code	

39. In what country do the following people currently live? (Tick the appropriate boxes)

	Deceased	Australia	New Z'land	USA	Canada	Fiji	Tonga	Samoa	Am. Samoa	Other, specify
(Code)	0	1	2	3	4	5	6	7	8	9
Spouse (00)										
Father (01)										
Mother (02)										
Father–in-law (11)										
Mother-in-law (21)										
Child 1 (31)										
Child 2 (32)										
Child 3 (33)										
Child 4 (34)										
Child 5 (35)										
Child 6 (36)										
Child 7 (37)										
Child 8 (38)										
Child 9 (39)										
Child 10 (40)										

40. Do any of them intend to move here?   Yes ☐   No ☐ → *Go to question 41*

Who?	Code	Why?	Code

41. Have you visited any of those overseas relatives in the past 12 months?   Yes ☐   No ☐

    Have you sent remittances to any?   Yes ☐   No ☐ → *Go to question*

        How much do you send per year?   In cash ☐☐☐☐☐☐

        In other forms (eg. goods, airtickets, etc)   ☐☐☐☐☐☐

    Do you know what it was used for?   Yes ☐   No ☐

        What was the money used for? _____

        _____ ☐☐

42. How often do you speak (phone) to relatives overseas?

Code		
1	Weekly	☐
2	Monthly	☐
3	Annually	☐

43. Do you intend to return to your 'home country', to live there permanently, at some time in the future?

Code		
1	No	☐
2	Don't know	☐
3	Yes	☐

Do you think you will return within one or five years? (Tick whichever is applicable)

Within	No	Code	Maybe	Code	Yes	Code
1 year	☐	1	☐	2	☐	3
5 years	☐	1	☐	2	☐	3

44. If you think you might leave, or intend to leave, why is that?
(Tick as many boxes as you consider relevant but also indicate the 3 most important, numbering them "1", "2" and "3")

Code	Reason for leaving	
		☐
01	Lack of close relatives/friends in this country	☐
02	Unemployed, can't find work	☐
03	Poor job, low pay, poor working conditions	☐
04	Don't get along with boss or co-workers	☐
05	Work contract or visa in this country will expire	☐
06	Poor schools, lack of schools	☐
07	Will complete training, studies or degree in this country	☐
08	Don't like community of residence, different values	☐
09	Family problems here	☐
10	High cost of living	☐
11	High crime rate	☐
12	Poor physical environment	☐
13	Don't like climate	☐
14	Language problems	☐
15	Visa problems	☐
16	Discrimination	☐
17	Political persecution, fear of political persecution	☐
18	Religious persecution, fear of religious persecution	☐
20	Other, specify_____	☐

Where would you like to go?_____ ☐☐

Why would you like to go to this country? _____

_____ ☐☐

45. What kind of job would you like there? _____ ☐☐

46. What changes, if any, in your home country or here, would encourage you to return there?
    [Do not answer this if you answered 'Yes" to question 43]

    _____ ☐☐

47. If you intend to remain in this country why do you intend to remain?
    [Do not answer this if you answered 'Yes" to question 43]

Code		
01	Have a good job and satisfactory income	☐
02	Close relatives and friends are in this country	☐
03	Children settled here	☐
04	Schools are good/ education availability	☐
05	Good health care	☐
06	Have successful business here	☐
07	Have good house	☐
08	Have nice neighbourhood and neighbours	☐
09	Freedom from political persecution	☐
10	Low level of crime	☐
11	Low cost of living	☐
12	Many social activities and things to do	☐
20	Other, specify	☐

APPENDIX 2

NEWSPAPER ARTICLES

- Trading Post Issue # 673 Wednesday August 23 2001, page 3
- Trading Post Issue # 673 Wednesday August 23, 2001, Page 4, Letters to the editor
- *Sydney Morning Herald,* 2 August 2000:
- *Sydney Morning Herald,* 3 August 2000:

TRADING POST ISSUE #673 WEDNESDAY AUGUST 23 2001:

Page 3:

ni-Vanuatu pharmacist departs for 'greener pasture' by Royson Willie Vanuatu's only ni-Vanuatu qualified pharmacist, Andrea Garae, has left the country to take up employment overseas in Australia. Ms Garae who used to work at Vila Central Hospital is believed to be the only ni-Vanuatu who holds a degree in the field. It is not the first time for ni-Vanuatu professionals within the medical community to leave the country for greener pastures overseas. Just this year in March, ni-Vanuatu qualified radiologist, Barry Melve, left the country for Palau where he was offered a job at the Palau Central Hospital.

This trend of 'brain drain' within the medical sector of Vanuatu has made the Vanuatu Medical Association very concerned. The President of the Association, Dr Hensley Garae said Vanuatu is heading for a disaster if something is not done soon about the trend. He said one of the reasons ni-Vanuatu medical professionals leave the public health sector is because of poor salaries and allowances and also because they are not recognized. He said one way to recognize ni-Vanuatu specialists within the public health sector is to localise posts that are held by overseas technical advisers once their contract expires. "It is the responsibility of the government that when they train people, they should secure their job within the country and create an environment that will attract them. At the moment we cannot pretend that everything is okay. Obviously something is wrong somewhere and no one can deny that" Dr Garae said. He said that the country needs such specialists also because of legal medical issues. "People are beginning to know their rights and once they start suing, those are the experts (pharmacist, radiologists) we need is such legal medical arrise" Dr Garae said. It is understood that there are already at least 4 ni-Vanuatu health professionals on overseas contract. Dr Garae said there are possibilities that one or two ni-Vanuatu experts within the medical sector will be leaving Vanuatu because of better offers of employment overseas. And, according to him, 'brain drain' is becoming a dangerous trend.

TRADING POST ISSUE #673 WEDNESDAY AUGUST 23, 2001

Page 4: Letters to the Editor: Recruitment of expatriate doctors

Dear Editor,

Recruitment of expatriate doctors and the work of staff

I want to comment on the above in regards to Vila Central Hospital. On 7July 2001 I took my son to hospital in Vila following an accident. At the hospital I had to wait for 3 hours before the radiologist arrived and 3 and a half hours for a doctor. My son was on a drip and his breathing was assisted with tubes. The nurses were running around telephoning, looking for the driving and the radiologist. They pushed my son twice to the x-ray room but as it was unattended, they had to push him back to the emergency room twice. This situation really made me think about my son's condition and the way that the staff on-call were nowhere to be found. After the 3 and a half hour wait for the doctor to arrive I thought that I would be satisfied but I wasn't. The doctor was Chinese and didn't speak French, English or Bislama. I found it hard to talk with him. I read, I write, I speak English French and Bislama but the doctor could have been speaking German or Arab.

These are some points which I don't agree with:

- The doctor didn't visit his patient for 3 days
- The doctor's absence made my family feel bad
- The doctor arrived very late
- The doctor couldn't speak one of the three languages of Vanuatu
- The radiologist on call was a football game
- Staff wasted time and money on calls and fuel because of these two men
- A man from Tanna (Paul) died as a result of adequate examination, treatment and care
- It seemed to me that Paul wasn't in a hospital but in Middlebush, Tanna (he cried, he called out, he felt terrible day and night, but I saw myself that he was not seen by an doctor
- Paul died at the hands of the careless Chinese doctor
- My son still does not walk well as a result of delayed treatment

The Government must seriously consider the recruitment of expatriate doctors (they must be professionals that know how to speak English, French or Bislama). Staff on call must be on standby at their homes and not at a football match or the beach. The Government must consider these points because when a minister, the president or prime minister is sick, they don't go to Vila central Hospital, they fly to Australia as they have money. But for us poor people of Vanuatu, we suffer until we die. It took me a month to find my son's medical report due to bad filing. I feel that most staff are only working for their salary and do not care about their job. Thank you for accepting action and support for this letter.

Tony Lulu, Efate.

SYDNEY MORNING HERALD, 2 AUGUST 2000:

Flight of doctors deals body blow to system

A frantic international search is under way to replace Indian Fijian doctors who have fled the unrest. **Malcolm Brown** *reports from Suva.*

The Fiji Ministry of Health will make an emergency trip to the Philippines later this month to recruit 48 doctors after five Indian Fijian doctors notified their intention to emigrate. More are to follow, and the nation's health system is approaching an abyss.

The country's director of hospital services, Dr Nacanieli Goneyali, one of those going to the Philippines, said the door was wide open for Australian doctors to fill the breach, but with salaries of only about $17,000 a year on offer, Fiji could not compete for their skills.

As a result, Fiji would turn to a developing country where the salary level was not such a problem.

The flight of Indian Fijian doctors, who say they no longer feel secure, is part of a larger brain-drain that has already seen the departure of nurses, teachers and accountants.

The Fiji Public Service Commission fears a collapse similar to that which occurred after the coups of 1987, when 67,000 Indians left Fiji, dealing the country a body blow from which it has barely recovered.

The chairman of the commission, Mr Sakeasi Waqanivavalagi, who will also seek to recruit public servants in the Philippines, said Fiji was losing many skilled workers every week.

"I don't know the exact number of vacancies but we are still receiving resignations and there will be more this week and next week," he said.

"I don't think the people behind this unrest gave any thought to the expected aftermath in terms of the brain-drain."

Four Australians who came to Fiji as public servants under the now partially suspended AusAID agreement have been removed as sanctions take effect.

Dr Goneyali said Fiji had a desperate time keeping doctors anyway, because of the better pay overseas.

In the past, Australia provided top-up salaries for Australian medical consultants but that had been terminated. Fijian investment in sending doctors overseas for postgraduate studies had backfired because the doctors, attracted by greater professional rewards, had not returned.

Last year the country initiated its own postgraduate training scheme for Pacific Island nations, funded by AusAID, but Australia's sanctions mean that is now threatened.

In the meantime, Fiji – with little more than 320 doctors, or one for about every 2,500 people – is struggling to provide basic services, and people in outlying areas are dying because they cannot get treatment routinely available in other countries.

At Vatukarasa village, near Sigatoka, in the west of Viti Levu, a 16-year-old girl failed to get the right diagnosis for a fever in February and died a week later in hospital. At Nayawa village, also in the west, a youth died of pneumonia because he could not get treatment in time.

Australian citizen Dr Norman Gage, who has lived in Fiji for two years after 20 years in private practice in Perth, said a potentially tragic result of the coup would be the winding up of the postgraduate medical schools.

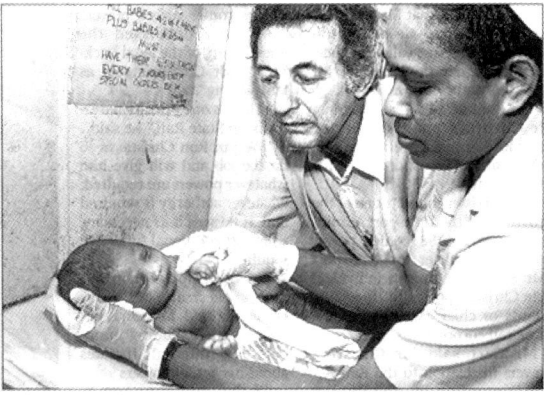

Staying on . . . expatriate Australian Dr Norman Gage is extending his Fijian contract for a year, despite taking a 12.5 per cent cut in pay. Photo: Brian Cassey

Dr Gage, head of Suva hospital's department of obstetrics and gynaecology, said it would probably be difficult to recruit teaching staff, and there had already been three resignations from the school of medicine's anatomy department.

Fiji was a challenge for a Western-trained doctor, he said, because many of its services were well behind modern developments. Pathology standards matched what he had seen in South Africa and Zimbabwe 30 years ago.

"You see huge complications from diseases common in Europe in the 19th century. Cancer of the cervix is commonest in the Pacific, but too many women come in when it is too serious and nothing can be done for them. We had a lady in last month who had a rare infection, leptospirosis, which is caused from rats that scuttle around the villages. She was coughing up blood. We put her in the intensive care unit for about 12 hours but she died."

Dr Gage, who has had a salary of about $40,000 a year but yesterday had to accept a 12.5 per cent pay cut imposed on the Fiji public service, said: "Doctors would have to come here for ideological reasons.

"But in Australia, you feel you're a cog in the wheel. Here, you feel special in a way that other people have not had the opportunity to be."

Dr Goneyali said a pool of available doctors would be created in the Philippines that could be called upon if the situation deteriorated.

Fiji had previously called on Chinese doctors, but there had been a language problem, he said.

After the 1987 coup, when Fiji had to call on the United Nations for help, many Burmese had come. He felt that eventually Fiji would have to turn to the UN again.

SYDNEY MORNING HERALD, 3 AUGUST 2000:

Yet another doctor gives up and packs his bags

EXODUS

Suva: Dr Bram Singh, 40, Fijian born and educated and a father of two, feels an enormous sense of upheaval as he prepares to migrate to Australia to set up in practice as a GP and gynaecologist.

"I have taken this course of action, well knowing that my plans were to stay here for the rest of my career," he said, readying himself for the move to Bundaberg, Queensland, in three weeks.

Dr Singh said that after the 1987 coups, the general perception among Indo-Fijians had been that things would improve, but since the May 19 coup attempt there had been fear and insecurity.

"It is not good enough to have

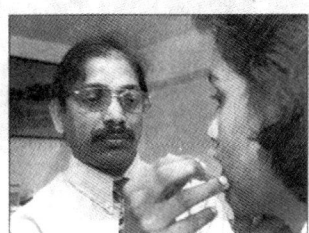

Dr Bram Singh is closing his general practice in Suva and moving to Queensland. Photo: Brian Cassey

all the money in the world and at the end of the day be worried you are going to be robbed or bashed," he said.

Dr Singh is one of a growing band of doctors, virtually all of Indian descent, who are moving to Australia, New Zealand, Canada and the United States. One of his colleagues, Dr Vijay Brahlad, moved to Brisbane last week.

Since the coup, most of Dr Singh's relatives – including both parents, two brothers and a sister – have settled in Brisbane.

Dr Singh saw the exodus of doctors after the coups of 1987. He stayed, but watched colleagues who had migrated establish themselves and prosper on higher incomes overseas.

"Over the years we have been able basically to improve the doctor situation in this country, though there have still been shortages," he said.

"The perception was that things were improving in Fiji. But if you saw Fiji on the day of the looting, May 19, you could see what the future might be.

"My assessment is that the police are not doing enough.

"I don't know whether it is because they are not in a position to do it or they don't want to do it because they have no commitment."

Dr Singh said he had heard of an Australian scheme for settling migrant doctors in areas of need and approached the Queensland branch of the Australian Medical Association, which told him there was a place available in Bundaberg.

"I am leaving with reluctance," he said.

"I have known the Fiji way of life. I would love to stay in Fiji, because when you are 40 you are well settled.

"I think there are a lot of doctors whose qualifications are being assessed for Australia, New Zealand, even the United States.

"As soon as they work this out, I think there will be a general exodus."

Malcolm Brown